It Is What It Is

A Memoir of Love & Loss

By Audrey Feldman

DEDICATED TO MY GERRY BOY...
AND TO THE WONDERFUL
FAMILY WE CREATED.

"It is what it is." The words my father spoke the night he was diagnosed with Stage IV Esophageal Cancer. The title of my mother's book. My parents. My heroes...

This book is a love story. The love of my parents for each other, and for all of us — their children and grandchildren, their siblings and their children and grandchildren, their friends.... My parents collected friendships through their many experiences, moves, jobs.... friendships which have survived the years. Even though my father is gone, he lives on in the memories of many, but most of all in the memories of my mother. A talented writer and lyricist, she has poured her talents into this memoir of the man she loved, the 56 years of their marriage, and their final struggle. They faced cancer as they faced everything else in life: together, and with grace and humor. They are people worth knowing, and this is a book worth reading.

It is what it is, and it is a wonderful tribute to a great and loving man and one of the most wonderful marriages I've ever seen.
SUSAN WYNN

It was early April 2007.
We were celebrating an early Passover Seder on a weekend when more of the family could go to my sister, Susan. During the evening my dad had some sort of attack. He had reflux disease and was used to heartburn; but this was different. It lasted too long and he was in severe pain. After a lot of Mylanta we talked a bit and I reassured my dad that it might be

an esophageal ulcer. It was treatable and easily diagnosed
by endoscopy. We talked a while longer which was not
unusual since I'm a talker and daddy, a great listener.
Dad (or poppy as I loved to call him) was one of my "go to
people". You know the kind; that special person or people
you can talk to about anything. They'll never judge you
even when you're wrong, too nervous about something, or
just need to vent. After that we hugged and returned to
the rest of the "fam". Mom and dad went to the hospital
where dad had his endoscopy and then they sent him for a
CAT scan on the same day. We were to hear the results on
April 20, 2007. I was awoken a little after 7 that morning
by a call from my then 17 year old son, Scott. He'd had a
car accident at the high school, was okay but...needless to
say I was there in a flash. I arrived on scene to see police,
2 smashed up cars and a couple of kids. After seeing
that everyone was unhurt we dealt with the cars. A very
cute young lady was the driver of the car my son literally
"bumped" into. Later that day through much texting,
Scott had his prom date.

We arrived home a few hours later. I started to make calls
to the insurance company and my son and I heard loud
popping and crackling sounds. Scott yelled the TV was
smoking. Sure enough our large 52 inch set was crackling,
smoking and ready to burst into flames. I disconnected
the plug from the outlet and called the township fire
marshal who told me to get everyone out of the house
immediately. I woke up my eldest son, Eric and the three of
us waited for the fire marshal to check my house. By this
time you can imagine that the feeling I was getting about
my dad was getting worse, so I did what any mother of 2
college kids who'd just gotten her son from an accident

and had the TV blow up do; I cried. They came and checked the house and luckily there would be no fire; not in my house anyway.

The phone finally rang late afternoon and my mom said that daddy had stage IV esophageal cancer which had spread to his stomach, liver and lungs. I was stunned. I expected the news to be bad but not this bad. I gathered my husband, Mark and kids downstairs and broke the news to them. I then called two of my dearest friends who came running to sit and cry with me. We were scheduled to see my niece's middle school show the next evening. I went out early since I planned to stay with my folks and assist with the oncology search. Mark and the boys arrived later in the day as they too adored daddy.

I saw mom and dad on April 21 and gave many hugs and said many "I love you's" We went to Andrea's show that night and she was amazing. I then did another "Ronni" move and sat in between my mom and dad during the show holding their hands and holding them in my heart. My mom tells their love story in typically "Audrey" fashion. She's witty, clever and downright funny. Our eternal optimist to the end; family and friends would call me up just to ask "so how is he really"? You see this is mom's way. She believes everything will be all right. She's to the point; a woman of one liners. She and daddy complimented each other so well. First and only true loves since they met at 17 & 19. Daddy came first to mom and mommy always came first to daddy. My sisters and I were well loved but never once questioned their deep devotion to each other. Not the stuff of Hollywood movies but rather the everyday sticking together through thick and thin, showing each other respect kind. There was never an occasion where my sisters and I didn't wait for the dance where mom and dad would strut their stuff. They did a mean Lindy and we loved the face daddy would make as he listened to the music and danced with his favorite gal. But there was more. They were there for everyone who needed them. They would run for any family, any friend, any of their kids and grandkids. They raised us to care about others.

So, when my dad faced the greatest challenge of his life, they did it in "Audrey and Gerry" style. Dad said he would share this journey and so mom started posting on the Caring Bridge website. Mom never missed a day and still keeps up with it today more than two years since my dad's passing. We figure that if mom hadn't written her journal entries with humor and optimism no one would have read it as often as they did.(even if they couldn't figure out how serious things were). My dad faced his death with courage, dignity and humor. He truly left me speechless (a hard thing for me). Dad had many side effects from the chemo and was unable to lift his own legs onto the bed. Mom did it every day. She'd let me help sometimes, but you see this was her sweetheart, her "Gerry boy".

I have the greatest love and affection for my parents. Their wisdom and humor help me to endure life's joys and sorrows. I told my mom to write a book worthy of Oprah or Ellen. I truly believe their story is inspiring and can demonstrate how ordinary people face life and death. As my sister Amy says on Caring Bridge-
"I love you mom and always dad".
RONNI MICHELSON

When I was a teenager living with my parents in what mom calls "Our Tenth Home," my dad asked me to go the store and buy some milk. I was in a lazy mood and didn't feel like it. I said to my dad "Why - what did you ever do for me?" I realized all too late that saying those words was a huge mistake and no matter how much I tried to apologize, dad wouldn't hear of it. He also didn't talk to me for 2 days. Dad and I would joke about it years later and it remained a joke until the end. However, I would like to share exactly what both my parents did for me.

It isn't until you live on your own that you realize what parents do. I'm not just talking about the basics (homes, food, clothes, etc.) They filled our lives with unconditional love. My dad instilled wisdom and my mom, the laughter. They both also handed down their very strong work ethic. Audrey actually reminds me of Lucy in "I Love Lucy." Growing up with my parents, you could see just how much dad loved mom. They were inseparable. When mom went to work at the same company as him, so many people wondered how they could spend so much time together. They obviously didn't know my parents. If my dad wasn't in a good mood, that would quickly change because of my mom's sense of humor. The love they had for each other was given to their children and of course, the grandchildren ten-fold. I love you mom and always dad!
AMY HANSEN

This book is divided into two sections:
the first 56 years and the last eight months.

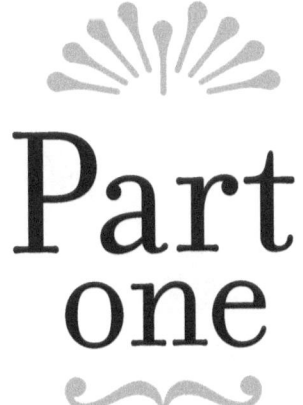

Part
one

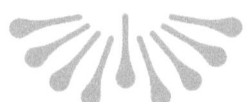

The first 56 years

Can I Play the Field?

It started at my brother Joel's Bar Mitzvah reception
in May of 1950. My detective cousin had to work that
night, leaving an empty seat at the young adult table. My
father asked a friend if he knew any families with single
sons to "fill in" for the night. Gerry was available on the
condition that he could play the field. I was standing
at the entrance to the ballroom, greeting the guests,
when a young man walked through the back doorway. I
thought he was the photographer's helper. Turned out to
be my Gerry, who returned home that night and told his
parents that he met the girl he was going to marry. Thus
begins our love story.

Hello, Baby!

I was a freshman at NYU, living in the Judson dorm.
There was a "community" phone in the hallway, and
every night the phone would ring and it was Gerry
saying, "Hello, Baby!" I'm not sure who he was trying to
emulate. Maybe Bogart? After a month, whichever girl
answered the hall phone would call to me and say, "Hello
Baby is on the phone." My roommate Claire came from
RD 2 in Englishtown, NJ… chicken farm country. Her
beau Marty used to come in to the city and we started
double dating. And we've double dated ever since.

THE PROPOSAL

After dating for three months, Gerry came out to our
Spring Valley home for the weekend and brought my
mother a house gift: a lovely ceramic pickle dish. We
went out that evening to a local restaurant and Gerry
proposed. I was 17. He was 19 (we did things differently
in those days). I came home from our date, went into
my parents' bedroom and said, "Gerry asked me to
marry him. What do you think?" My mother said,"
Well, he's a great guy and it's O.K. with us, but if you
don't marry him, I'm not giving back the pickle dish!"
This is romantic? Joel said,"I love him, I love him!",
and Gerry was Joel's big brother from that day on.

EVELYN -THE MOTHER-IN-LAW

When I accepted the proposal, Gerry wanted me to
meet the parents. I heard that his mother was very
active in organizations and loved to bake. So I decided
to get her something very special for the occasion.
Went to Greenwich Village and bought a beautiful
organdy hostess apron, hand-painted with her name
on it. We walked into their home, I gave her the special
gift and she threw it back at me saying, "You know I
sew. Why would you give me something I can make
myself?" That was one of her kinder comments. For
years I searched for somebody named Evelyn so they
could enjoy the beautiful apron. Finally threw it away!
At this time in our relationship, Evelyn decided she did
not want me as a daughter-in-law, and offered Gerry
$10,000 plus a Cadillac not to marry me. He thought

it was a rather disingenuous offer. First of all, he had no intention of letting me go. Secondly, he knew if he said yes to the offer, she would have told him he had no character, and would have rescinded the "bribe." But the in-law meeting was not all terrifying. I also met Gerry's father, Max…a dignified, loving man who was always welcoming. Luckily, Gerry Boy inherited his father's genes. Must be true that opposites attract!

The Thing About the Ring

I was vacationing in Atlantic City with my parents and brother, Joel. Gerry told them he was coming out for the weekend and was going to surprise me with an engagement ring. Everybody knew but me. We walked into the dining room to our assigned table and everyone around us was filled with excitement. I sat down and noticed a white oval on my plate. I said to Gerry, "Where's your egg?" It took me a few seconds to realize the "egg" was a box containing my beautiful ring. As Homer Simpson would say, DOH!

The Unsurprise Shower

My next door neighbor was throwing the "surprise" bridal shower. I was up late the night before, decorating. I also gave her the guest list and planned the menu. Then I practiced all day trying to look surprised. Think I pulled it off!

THE WEDDING

After 6 months of preparation, the Big Day arrived.
March 4, 1951. It was held at the Riverside Plaza Hotel
in New York City. I was in the elevator en route to the
ceremony with Gerry, both sets of parents, my brother
and a few relatives. The door opened and there was
a group waiting for the next elevator, including Gerry's
Brooklyn friends in the wedding party. Evelyn pointed
to one of the girls and said, "That's the girl he
should have married!" The doors slowly closed, but
our mouths were all open... not quite believing
what we just heard.

Let's get to the good part. Leibele Waldman and the
Sterner choir sang during our ceremony. It was like
an opera! During the dinner, my dad Irving sang
"Always." Irving had a beautiful tenor voice
that became more beautiful after a few drinks, and we
had quite a few toasts that night.

I sang "My Foolish Heart," our special song. Gerry's
little cousin Mimi danced around in her special gown,
fashioned by her mom, Aunt Irene. Ekka (my mom's
nickname, since she couldn't pronounce Esther when
she was little) did her famous belly dance. Gerry's
brother Stan and his bride of one year, Dolores, were in
our wedding party. Brother Joel, who was about 5'4" at

the time, was not in the wedding party. One year later, the little shrimp was over 6 feet tall. My roommate Claire was one of my maids of honor, and two months later, I was her matron of honor.

Evelyn was so busy running around complaining about everything, that she missed most of the photo shoots. Years later, Gerry wanted to hang up a picture of his father, but the only nice one was of Gerry walking down the aisle with both parents. On my wall is a framed picture of Gerry and his dad. It's amazing how you can get rid of a disturbing presence with scissors.

THE HONEYMOON

Since we were so young, we listened to all the advice from our elders. Go to Florida by train. It's cheaper than flying. Stay at a hotel across the street from the beach. It's cheaper. Bad advice, but we had a wonderful time in spite of it. We went into a restaurant for dinner one night, and the waitress looked at the two "kids" at her table and asked if we'd like some hamburgers. Indignantly, we ordered steak… the most expensive on the menu. We may have been kids, but we were married ones.

FIRST HOME

I was now 18, Gerry was 20 and we were homeowners
in Spring Valley, NY. A lovely brick ranch in a lovely
neighborhood. We had a housewarming, and when
I started introducing someone to Evelyn, I couldn't
remember her last name. "This is my mother-in-law,
Mrs. Uh... uh... uh". She icily reminded me that her
last name was the same as mine. Oops! Gerry, the new
property owner, became obsessed with security. He
locked the front door, the side door, the back door,
and then rechecked them a few times before he could
finally sleep securely. Took my driving test the day my
in-laws were coming for a visit. Her visits generally
unnerved me. So, I tried to start the car with my
house keys. I tried to parallel park and hit the cars in
front and in back. When the test was over, I asked the
instructor if I passed. He said, "Passed? I'm glad I'm
alive!" By the way, I did pass the second one.

Gerry's friend Mike used to drive out from the Bronx
and would bring all his current girl friends for our
approval. One very fancy girl got a very un-fancy tour
of our house. When we were on the way downstairs
to see the basement, the rack that was on the door
(holding mops, brooms, etc) broke...and the cleaning
supplies fell on her. She wasn't his girl friend for long.
Then one day he brought Carol, and it was a done deal.
They were married and we were friends forever after.

In November of 1951, Phil and Bev (Gerry's old school friends) were married. Those were the days when babies got married and grew up with their babies.

I still remember one particular fetish of mine as a young bride. I kept all the tags on the bed pillows and decorative pillows, tucking them in when company was coming. Gerry asked me why I didn't just cut them off, and I told him, "I can't. It says Don't remove under penalty of law." Gerry started shaking his head in bewilderment, and kept shaking it for 56 years.

FIRST BABY

Our beautiful Susan was born in June of 1952. By the time she was two months old, Gerry and I were 22 and 20. Getting on in years. When she was 8 months old, I cut her bangs. She looked so cute, I wrote a poem which I sent to Mamie Eisenhower (wife of our prez), who also sported bangs. Poem follows:

As first lady of the nation you have caused quite a sensation
With your bangs that look so charming and so sweet.
And as most the young and fair do like to imitate your
hair-do I just couldn't let my daughter miss the treat.
So I took my little cutie, eight months old and quite a beauty
And I combed the silken hair down past her eyes
And the darling started crying as my steady hand kept trying
To cut off the right amount despite her sighs.
Well, she fussed so with the new cut
that it looks more like a crew cut
But we're proud of the effect upon her dome
For we can't help but compare a certain title you both share.
Little Susan is First Lady in our home.

I did get an answer from the White House! A lovely card from Mamie Eisenhower's secretary.

One day we decided to get a collie. Shep was a tri-colored dog and really lovable. To us. The mailman was afraid to come to the door and my father used to wave to us from the street until we tied her up. She finally got used to people and we decided it was time to invite the in-laws for a visit to meet their new granddog. We put the puppy outside with a bowl of water and tied him to the railing. Wanted to introduce him to Evelyn gradually. Finally took the mother-in-law outside to meet our gorgeous Shep, and all we saw was a mangy looking, mud-covered hound. It seems he knocked the water bowl over and rolled in the mud. Shep had a great time. Evelyn was horrified. Shep had fun roaming the neighborhood and bringing toys home that he found in the backyards. We had to ring all the doorbells to return the stuff, since we had no idea where our dog burglar stole it from. Sometimes the doorbell would ring, and the kids would say, "Can Shep come out and play?" Speaking of our pooch, one day our grouchy next-door neighbor rang our bell and started screaming at us. It seems that Shep made a pit stop on his lawn, and he stepped in it. Gerry, usually sweet and agreeable, surprised me when he answered the neighbor with, "I hope you were barefoot."

At 8 months old, Susan said her first word: shit. Then she said her second word: oh. Sometimes she said them together: oh, shit! (don't know where she could have heard that). I then started watching my language. My mother taught her how to say Dodgers (dadas). So she had a three word vocabulary "oh shit dadas". In the baby book, I wrote that her first word was mama. Shep used to sleep under Susan's crib and never left her side. One day we noticed that Susi was having trouble breathing. Unfortunately, she was allergic to the dog, so Shep went to a new home. And so did we. We were living in Spring Valley for two years, 15 minutes from my folks, but Gerry commuted to Brooklyn every day... home of the family children's sleepwear business. After much discussion, it was decided that we should move closer to work, so we set about looking for a new home.

Our Second Home

Found a great split level in East Meadow, NY. We became involved with our local Temple's theatre group, where I wrote and acted in the plays and Gerry stage-managed. It's amazing what you can do when you're young. I still remember one of the lyrics I wrote (with apologies to South Pacific):

Some detectives they are thin, Some detectives they are fat
Some detectives smoke a pipe and wear a
Sherlock Holmes-type hat
You can find them in the city or out in the country sticks.
What don't we like? We don't like dicks.

Gerry had stage managing down to a science. Everything went like clockwork. In one show, I decided to give him a line on stage. After all his work, I wanted him to be recognized. We sang:

This is our once a year day, once a year day, it's our once a year for certain.
This is our once a year day, once a year day...
(and Gerry ran onstage, with arms waving and sang):
Once a year I pull the curtain!

I became pregnant in July of 1954. One kid and one on the way and I still couldn't vote. Wasn't 21 until August. Since we didn't know the area too well, I asked my uncle, a Nassau County detective, if he knew anything about Nassau Hospital in Minneola. His reply: "Good morgue." That's not exactly what I wanted to hear. We now had a front door, side door and garage door, and Gerry kept up his vigil every night, making sure the doors were locked and his family protected.

SECOND BABY

Gave birth to our Ronni in April of 1955. We originally planned to name her Robin, but she weighed in at 8 pounds, 10-1/2 ounces...too big for a Robin, and decided to name her Ronni. Her middle name is Jo (Little Women). Named her after 2 grandmothers and needed R and J. She didn't forgive us for years for giving her 2 boy's names, especially when she was in high school and they wanted to know why she was cutting boy's gym class . She even got offers to join the Air Force!

It was such fun having two gorgeous little girls. I'd play-act all the musicals with them and they loved Peter Pan. Susan was Wendy and Ronni was Peter Pan. At this time I started writing songs, and my dad had a connection with Republic Music Corp through Lee Eastman, a business associate and father of Linda Eastman (Paul McCartney's wife). Once a week I'd leave the kids with a baby sitter and take the train to New York to peddle my latest stuff. Met with a wonderful man named Bugs Bower who arranged "Catch a Falling Star" for Perry Como. He made many demo records, and we came close a few times, but something always got in the way. Teresa Brewer was supposed to do one of my songs. She was in California, song session was in New York and shazam! There was an airplane strike. By time she got to New York, they were on to other projects, and my big chance of stardom was squelched.

Back to motherhood. I remember one particular day when the front door bell rang. I went outside and there was Susan with a doll carriage and a large doll, dressed in fancy doll clothes and a big bonnet. The face on the doll seemed familiar. It took me a few seconds to realize the "doll" was actually Ronni. Yes, it was a strange and eerie feeling. They really got me!

And then, Bingo! I was pregnant again!

Third Baby

Amy arrived in February of 1957, two days after a blizzard. So glad she waited to make her debut. Now we were the parents of three gorgeous girls. Some stupid people would come up to Gerry and offer him sympathy for having another girl. He wouldn't have it any other way. He loved his girls and they sure loved him. As soon as Amy could crawl around, her sisters included her in their musical performances. Susan was still Wendy. Ronni was still Peter Pan. And Amy, thrilled to be with her big sisters, was either Captain Hook, the alligator, or everybody else! Ronni had a habit of taking her clothes off, and one day she walked in naked and bent down near Amy the Alligator. The alligator, in true method acting mode, bit her in the butt.

Complaint Poetry

After buying more than one product of inferior quality, I decided to complain to the manufacturers. Wrote to one cosmetics firm about a nail file: "You said a lifetime guarantee. In this you kept your trust. The stainless steel's still going strong, but the handle bit the dust." The president called me at work to say that he never wrote a poem before, but he wanted to reply in due fashion, and had to let me hear it before it was mailed out. That was such fun! Complained about an instant cereal many years ago. Thought it tasted like a mouthful of sand. The company apologized and sent me one dozen boxes of the same crap I complained about. Guess they meant well.

Evelyn's Birthday Gifts

I would try to pick out a suitable gift every year, and every year I would get it back. One year I gave up on the gift idea and decided to give a charitable donation in her honor. Got that back, too. "What do you mean by giving something in my name? I'm not dead yet!" (That reminds me of a song from Spamalot). Then a great idea hit me. If I needed a blue purse, I'd give it to her, knowing I'd go home with it. Thereafter, every birthday I'd get what I wanted for myself and the mother-in-law from hell got the satisfaction of tossing it back.

The Intruder

Gerry used to visit brother Stanley and sister-in-law Dolores in Lynchburg, VA. That's where the manufacturing plant was for our sleepwear business. On one visit, Gerry was sleeping on the couch in the living room when he heard a noise. He then thought he heard footsteps. He figured if he kept still and didn't move, whoever was in the house wouldn't know he was there. And then suddenly the dining room light went on and a man was walking around. Gerry jumped off the couch and started screaming, "What are you doing here? STANLEY!" No sound from Stanley's room. Gerry pushed the man out of the front door, ran into Stan's bedroom and said, "Where were you? I was calling you. Someone broke into the house!" Stanley thought he was dreaming. So he called the police, Dolores got up and put up a pot of coffee and the police car arrived. They were all sitting around answering questions and sipping java, when one of the policemen said, "We have someone in the car. Would you like to identify him?" This guy was sitting in the car for over twenty minutes. Gerry identified him, but did not press charges. It seems that the intruder was very drunk, looking for his girlfriend and he picked the wrong house. While he was walking down the street, he saw the police car with lights flashing and hailed it. He thought it was a cab.

Our Third Home

Gerry used to make so many business trips to Lynchburg, it was decided that we should move there. So we sold our home in East Meadow and moved to non-Yankee country. Cousins Marion and Aaron made us a farewell party, and I still remember the note on Aunt Rudy's gift (she was Ekka's oldest sister): "Dear Audrey and Gerry. We hate to see you." She forgot to write the word "GO".

After the episode of the break-in at Stanley's house, Gerry ran up and down the stairs of our new home a few extra times a night, making sure all the doors were locked. Took a while before the Virginians could understand my dialect and I understood what they were saying. Rapid New York accent versus slow Southern drawl. But we adapted and loved living there.

Natural Bridge, one of the Seven Wonders of the World, was not too far away, so all of our visitors had to see it. Come to think of it, I can't remember why it was such a wonder!

I took the girls with me once a week to perform musical therapy at the Lynchburg Training School, a facility for the medically and mentally disabled. The patients loved the girls (thought they were living dolls), and held them on their laps while we sang their favorite songs. When you talk about the "War" in Virginia, there was only one: The Civil War. One patient declared, "My granddaddy was in the War." I said, "That's wonderful!" And she proudly replied, "Yep, he was a deserter!"

It Seems Like Yesterday...

We had a parakeet named Polly. Then a dear friend gave us a Siamese cat that we named Sheba. For months, Sheba would sit on the arm of the sofa, staring at the bird cage. On a day that Gerry went out to play golf for the first time, Sheba lunged at the cage, the door opened and Polly flew out. I managed to throw a towel over Polly and retrieve her before Sheba ate her for dinner. Everything returned to normal, and Gerry walked in with his golfing buddy. They were covered in mud and scored the highest score ever recorded. It seems they found every mud trap, and this was Gerry's first and last game of golf.

My folks visited quite often, and one day we took them to Thomas Jefferson's Home, Monticello, in Charlottesville. Ekka walked in, took one look at the main parlor and said, "Oh, what I could do with this room!" She loved to rearrange furniture, but we told her this was a no-no. Ekka's sister Bernice lived in Charlottesville, along with her clan, so we had Rofheart family nearby, always a plus.

Another memory that stays in my mind is the skyline view of Lynchburg as you entered the city. A prominent landmark was the Hotel Virginia, proudly lit up with large neon letters. As the letters wore out, they never bothered to change the bulbs, and eventually the sign read: "Hot Virgin."

Southern Entertaining

The going rage was a large theme party once a year, and many dinner parties and luncheons throughout the year. Dolores and I would host dinners together many times, and we knew that southern ladies despised instant coffee. So we made instant coffee, poured it into a percolator and got rave reviews on our culinary expertise. We once hosted a luncheon at a restaurant, and wanted to do something different. We told them to add spinach to the rice for a nice flavor. What we didn't consider was the outcome. We served ugly green rice, and although the taste was O.K., it looked horrible!

Gerry and I hosted a witch party one year (the year of the Kennedy/Nixon election). We made posters of all the candidates in witch costumes and the guests outdid themselves with creativity. Still remember one couple arriving as a sand-witch! Stan and Dolores had a Hawaiian luau one time. I was going to be a hula dancer and Gerry a beach bum. At the last minute, we changed costumes and Gerry was the hula dancer and I was the beach bum. It was sort of funny and we were young enough to be dopey! When you had the once-a-year theme party, the host usually invited and cooked for over 100 people. We had tables (cutting tables from our factory), but never enough chairs. So we called the local funeral parlor and they delivered all the chairs and picked them up the next day. Good advertising for them, but looking back, it was a little ghoulish

Troubled Times

While we were living in the South, desegregation began. The pool we took our girls to for swimming lessons was told to integrate. So they closed the pool. The stores had white drinking fountains and colored drinking fountains. As a New Yorker, I found it all sickening. I remember going to a lunch counter, and a black man was sitting there all alone. I sat down next to him and they asked me what I wanted. I said, "He was here first." They totally ignored him and asked me again. I told them in a very loud voice, "He was here first. I'll wait." They served him because they had to, and I couldn't understand what all the fuss was about. It was just the way we were all brought up. I never knew about segregation and they never knew about integration. Just as we were settling into our Southern lifestyle, the family business started going downhill, and we were told to move back to New York. Before we moved back, we had one more party, a Mocktail Party for our girls. All the neighborhood kids came dressed in their parents' clothes, and we served punch and snacks and they looked so darling!

Our Fourth Home

Moved back to Spring Valley, into my parents' home, until we could figure out our future. The girls went to the same school I went to as a young girl and Gerry commuted to his office in Brooklyn (déjà vu...that's how we started). One day Ekka spent hours making kreplach (little meat dumplings). She put this delicacy on the kitchen counter to cool, came in an hour later and all the kreplach were gone. And Sheba was sitting on the counter, licking her lips. Guess her cooking was the cat's meow!

An aside about my parents. Ekka was like Auntie Mame, a beatnik/hippie way ahead of her time. She was proud of the fact that she was one of the first to wear a one-piece short bathing suit to the beach. The fashion mode at that time was a two-piece set with long bloomers. The police chased her into the ocean and made her stay there until everyone left the beach. They considered her indecent. This talented lady studied dance at Chalif's famous Russian ballet school in the twenties, and was in the corps de ballet at the Roxy Theater in New York City (part of the Roxyettes). Ekka's maiden name was Rofheart. Her parents built a group of 16 bungalows in Rockaway, but six were washed away in a tidal wave. Most of the ten remaining bungalows were rented by the grown Rofheart kids for the summer, so all the cousins grew up with fond memories of the beach. Years later the cousins formed the Rofheart Family Circle: Marion and Aaron, Betty Anne, Bobbie and Ronnie, Arnold and Harriet, Ruth, Alan and Bess, Jane and Barry, Joel and Diane. Arnold was the president because he was the only one with the last name of Rofheart.

Irving started life as a young kid on the East Side of New York. Coming from a large, poor family, he did what he could to help bring in money. He sold newspapers on the subway when he was ten years old, and sold milk to the tenement neighbors by dipping a ladle into a large container of milk, running up 6 flights of stairs and selling the ladle of milk for a nickel. He never had the chance to go to high school, but was a self-taught, brilliant man, who was a realtor in New York City for many years. Most of his spare time was spent in doing charity and volunteer work. He figured that if you made it up the ladder, you always had to reach your hand out to help someone else succeed.

This helping-hand philosophy has carried down to his children, grand children and great grandchildren. What a great gene to possess! He lost most of his siblings at an early age, but his surviving sister, Sadie, had one daughter, Selma, who became my mentor...and more of a sister than a cousin.

Before the Home Decorating Channel

One day Ekka and I decided to put up wall paper. There was a new product out called Trimz. All you had to do was soak it in the bathtub, carry the dripping paper through the house and stick it to the wall. It was pre-pasted. We put up a wall of ivy in the dining room, and were so very proud of ourselves. My dad, Irving, sat across from the wall every night and never noticed it! Then a neighbor came in to look at our handiwork, and said, "You know....you're supposed to cut the directions off the end before you paste it." So for many years, the dining room wall had ivy and how-to directions hanging on it.

Our Fifth Home

We read all the real estate rentals in the New York Times and found a great apartment in Riverdale, NY: Three bedrooms, 2 baths and a terrace overlooking the pool in the back. Here we go again. First thing we did was screen in the terrace so Sheba couldn't escape, and Gerry didn't have to worry about locking the back door. Met new friends and started out in the North again.

Amy still had a southern accent . The kids started new schools (again). Susan came home and showed me a piece of paper with her address on it. It said "3950 Blackstone Avenue, Bronx, NY." I thought she made a mistake. Got the apartment from an ad in the Times and it explicitly said "Riverdale." Went to school, spoke to the teacher and discovered that I lived in the Bronx!

I wrote a show as a school fundraiser called "Riverdale on the Rocks" and met my future collaborator, Don Freeberg. He wrote music and I wrote lyrics. Don was a member of the BMI Workshop in New York City, directed by Broadway musical director Lehman Engel. Don arranged for me to have an audition and I aced it. We wrote music and lyrics to scores of shows, including Chayefsky's "Marty." There were a few people in our workshop who made it big time. Bob Brittan wrote "Raisin" and Ed Kleban wrote the lyrics to "A Chorus Line." But Paddy Chayefsky wasn't ready to turn Marty into a musical at that time. When he finally decided to hear our songs, he suddenly passed away and we put Marty on hold. Many years later, someone else obtained the rights and we're still sitting with the most wonderful Broadway show never to be seen. Later on, Don brought his friend's son into the workshop who had better luck than we did. His name is Alan Menken (Little Mermaid, Beauty and the Beast, etc.).

While we were living there, Ekka and Irving decided to move to a building a block away from us. They missed their kids and grandkids so much, they left Spring Valley. We belonged to the Riverdale Jewish Center, and one day I was asked to write a series of 4 scripts for a TV program called "The Jewish 4th R." Ekka did the choreography, I did the narration and Susan and Ronni were in the chorus. Before the 4th program aired, an event occurred that took all programming off the air. Kennedy was assassinated. Time stopped for every one. I'm sure you all remember where you were when you heard the news.

LET'S GO CAMPING

It all started when my brother Joel, his wife and 10-month old baby Ethan visited from Colorado. Joel said, "You want to go camping?" We figured, why not? Drove to North Truro, Massachusetts. Joel figured it was a four hour drive. It was actually 9 hours away. We set up the tent in the dark and were starving!!! A neighbor offered us his dying embers to cook some dinner, and we went to sleep exhausted. The next morning, I went outside and looked at the tent site. Ours looked like Tobacco Road. I asked my brother if it was supposed to be so lop-sided and he said, "Oh, this is first time I ever set up a tent." And we thought he was a pro.

Had such a good time, though, that we and three other families decided to seriously try camping. Bought tents and all the gear. Had eleven kids between us and evenings were spent singing around the camp fire, while the kids' sneakers dried out, suspended from tree branches. Went to Rudd Pond in upstate New York on Memorial and Labor Day weekends, and spent July 4th week in Cape Cod. In Rudd Pond we walked out of the tent one day to discover Ronni swinging on a tree limb over the lake. She had more guts than we did. One day Gerry took the kids fishing. Ronni caught something called a crappie (tasted better than it sounded). It was the size of a sardine. I had to cook it and divide it into 5 portions. We each had one bite (and it was good).

Should mention that Gerry's love of fishing began when he was very young. His Uncle Bob took Gerry and big brother Stan fishing in the ocean off Long Beach, NY. If they didn't have any bites, Bob would pour beer into the water to try to get the fish drunk, saying, "Time to eat!" Another fish story shows how optimistic Gerry was. Stan and his friend bought an outboard motor. They would rent a rowboat in the cold winter days, attach the motor and go fishing for flounder. When Gerry was about twelve years old, they offered him a proposition he couldn't resist. If he paid for one third of the motor, he could go fishing with them. He was overjoyed! He was even given the honor of sitting in the rumble seat, holding the motor with his frozen hands. When they got to the beach, they also allowed him to push the boat off into the icy water, and he loved every minute of it!

After a few years of camping in one large tent, we set up pup tents so the girls could bring their friends. Only downside was walking through the woods to use the bathroom. The guys really had the advantage. I remember footsteps running past the tent one night and finally a woman's voice yelling at her dog, "This is the last time I take you camping!"

OUR SIXTH HOME

There was an apartment a few blocks away that caught our eye. A beautiful place at 3777 Independence Avenue in Riverdale (the Bronx). It was sort of a fancy building and I don't think some of the tenants were too pleased when we brought cartons over on dollies, with the help of our friend Marvin. I got a job as a sales lady in a clothing store nearby. Problem was, I was not good at lying. When one customer walked out of the dressing room, preening, I said, "Mrs. Harris, what can I say?" Couldn't tell a short, plump woman that she looked "fabulous" in a tight knit dress. I met one of the customers in our building lobby one day and she wanted to know what I was doing in HER building. When I told her I lived there, she was bummed. She

didn't have to worry for long. Just as we were settling
into our new home, our family business went bottoms
up. Gerry's dad, Max, founded the company and during
the decades, employed many of his siblings and their
children, as well as his two sons. He was more upset
about the family losing jobs than he was about losing
his life's work.

Gerry drove a limousine for a while. He drove people
into New York City 5 days a week and on weekends
he drove them to hotels in the mountains…not a
very satisfying way to make a living when they all
complained about which one should be dropped off
first. He finally landed a job in the garment business,
and we planned a house warming for a Saturday
night. The night before the party, Gerry came home
to announce that he had been fired. It seems that
the people who hired him wanted the rights to our
company's name, which was a very popular one years
ago. As soon as they got the name, they got rid of the
name giver. So, we had the party anyway, and nobody
knew it was a good bye party (except our friend Marvin
and his wife Arlene).

We started off with everything and ended up with nothing – except the most important thing of all: each other and our kids. Got a 2 bedroom, 1 bath apartment on Sadore Lane in Yonkers, NY. The kids started new schools again. It was very cramped there and our bedroom window overlooked a fire escape. One day in a self-pitying mood, I said, "This place looks like a tenement. All we need is laundry hanging outside." When I walked out of the room, Gerry strung up a clothes line across the bedroom and hung laundry on it. Very smart guy. We had a good laugh and I never complained again. I do remember one day when Amy told me she saw a mouse in the kitchen. I told her not to be ridiculous. We didn't have mice! A few minutes later, I went to my bedroom closet, put on my bathrobe, put my hand in my pocket, and you guessed it. A mouse jumped out. Don't recall if I screamed or changed my underwear, but we closed the room off and started swinging at the critter with a broom and it disappeared into nowhere. Never saw it again!!!

We were there a few months when I opened a local paper and saw in 24 point bold letters a headline saying, "Feldman Goes Bankrupt." When our Lynchburg factory closed, we had to file a substantial bankruptcy claim. People would stop me in the super market and say, "Are you the Feldman from the paper?" I would hold my head up high and proudly say, "Yup!" Gerry found another job in the garment

business with wonderful, honest people, but we still
needed additional income. I knew I had to get a job, but
didn't know what I was qualified for. The only other
time I worked was when we lived in Lynchburg and
I became a buyer in a department store. I might add
that when we left Lynchburg, I owed the store more
money than I ever earned. Couldn't resist all the new
stuff that came in. A friend suggested that I become
a copywriter. Good idea! Saw an ad in the paper and
went for an interview. Problem was, I didn't know what
a copywriter was. I just figured that if I could write
plays and lyrics, I could write anything. They asked
me if I brought my portfolio. I told them I left it home.
Actually, I didn't know what a portfolio was! But I got
the job anyway. When they asked me if I could do TV
scripts, I said, "Of course." Then I came home, called
my friend Gary Franklin, who was a TV drama critic,
and asked him to clue me in on things I never heard of.
A "TCU" was a tight close-up, for instance.

I figured you learn by doing, and I learned a lot. I wrote
the copy for packaging and ads and my friend Lee did
the art work. When he was too busy to finish all his
projects, he would ask me to help, and I learned to
do silk screen separations. Remember, this was way
before computers. I had the title of public relations
director. One time I got a phone call, and the person
on the other end asked me if there were a lot of people
in my department. I said,"You're talking to her. Just
me." My boss was walking past and overheard the

conversation and did I get hell. " You never tell people that. You have to pretend that this is a very big operation, and there are dozens of people in your department." I did the work of dozens of people and if I recall, I made $5.00 an hour. Gerry was hired by a very prestigious lingerie company and everything was coming up roses, so we did what we did best. We decided to move to larger quarters.

Our Eighth Home

A few blocks down the road on Central Avenue in Yonkers was a complex called Westchester Towers. It was a beautiful, spacious apartment, and the first thing we did was screen in the terrace for Sheba. Shortly after we moved in, Ekka and Irving decided to move into the same building. Good thing we loved each other. We loved camping so much, we decided to trade in our tent for a pop-up trailer. We shlepped this trailer all over the place, even to Expo in Canada. Finally got tired of towing it, and parked it in a campground in northern New Jersey called Tall Timbers. Most weekends were spent there. When you're camping, time seems to stand still and you really relax... especially after cocktail hour. After a few years of camping without a bathroom, we traded the Pop-up in for a travel trailer. The kitchen table converted to a bed, the couch became a bed and there were double bunks over the couch, plus a kitchen and a bathroom. Happiness!!!

We moved to a camp site called Pleasant Acres, PAC for short. I thought PAC stood for Protestants and Catholics. Finally met 2 more Jewish families, but religion really doesn't matter when you're in the woods. Camping is the great equalizer.

While living here, Gerry's Dad passed away from cancer. He was a wonderful man, dearly missed by all. I remember one of his granddaughters at his funeral saying, "The wrong one went!" Yes, Evelyn was still around. She said horrible, ugly things to her granddaughters before the funeral, but at the chapel her demeanor changed. She pointed to the girls, saying, "Look at my beautiful flowers." Talk about method acting!I was still working as a copywriter, and when I came home from work one day, Gerry told me he had sold some stock. I was pissed off and told him that any important decisions should be discussed before acting on them. He got the message. A few months later I got a call at work. Gerry said, "You said we should discuss any important decisions." I agreed. He said, "I'm quitting my job." I told him to do whatever he had to do. We could always live in the trailer. When he walked into his boss's office to resign, they wouldn't hear of it. All of a sudden they started treating him with respect, so he decided to stay until he found another job.

When we lived here, we became involved with the Northeast Jewish Center theater group. I wrote or performed, the girls performed and Gerry was stage manager. We also had a hootenanny group and the kids strummed away for a few years, singing the latest folk songs (that was the time of "Blowin' in the Wind.") One day I started brushing my hair and my arm got stuck in the up position. Went to the doctor and was told I needed a shoulder revision. Both shoulders had arthritis, and we did the worst first (like the rhyme?). Took a year of therapy for each shoulder to get back full range of motion, and people kept telling me how sorry they were I couldn't play the guitar anymore. I tried to explain that I never played the guitar. My girls did. I just sang and occasionally tuned it. They didn't believe me. Gerry was offered a job with a Madison Avenue lingerie firm, where he remained for 25 years. His sterling reputation in the garment business grew more and more every year, and people knew who to go to in a crisis.

And one day the light bulbs went off in our heads. Why rent when we can buy?

You guessed it.

Found a beautiful condo in Hartsdale, NY called
High Point...still on Central Avenue, but 15 minutes
North. By this time, my folks moved to Florida, so
they didn't follow us. It was actually a 2 bedroom, 1-1/2
bath apartment, but it had a terrific layout, including
2 terraces. Gerry had to go out of town on business
the day before the move, so I directed the whole move.
Then I called in carpenters and told them to partition
the dining room area off to make a third bedroom.
We discussed this before Gerry's trip, but never
went into specifics. So I just told them to put the
wall here, put the folding door there, and shazam,
a third bedroom appeared.

Every time we moved, I made up special moving
notices. In this case I remember saying, "Just in case
you haven't heard, we're moving April 23rd." Got a call
from the builder a few weeks before the move saying
he wanted to change the date to April 24th. Normally, I
would have been cooperative, but let's face it. Nothing
rhymed with the 24th! So I ranted and raved and got
my date. Sheba started showing her age and died at
18 years old. Really missed this family member. Got
another Siamese named Snuggy and she turned out
to be the cat from hell. Gave her away ASAP. Then I
surprised Gerry with an Irish Setter that I found at
the pound. Her name was Samantha and we loved her.
Even took her camping in the trailer, where she

stretched out over the entire couch. But we worked all day and she was cooped up in small quarters all day and we realized she needed a home with people and space... where she could run around all day. Found a great family for her, and decided: No More Pets! Except for our parakeet named Pippin.

While we were there, Joel, Diane and their four kids came East for the summer and stayed at a place in the Hamptons. We visited them one weekend and Gerry decided to take all the kids fishing off the dock. They were gone for a few hours, and Gerry wouldn't leave until every kid caught a fish. Our girls, plus Ethan, Naomi and Simeon caught some early on, but little Andrea was still waiting. Finally, she hooked one, and the smiling fishermen brought back delicious fish for dinner.

While living here, we started celebrating Thanksgiving with Carol and Mike and their daughters, Ellen and Julie, at their home in Ardsley. One Thanksgiving, when everyone was seated at the dining room table, Carol, Gerry and I went into the kitchen to get the turkey (uncarved, luckily) and fixings. A glass dropped out of an upper cabinet, broke and shattered all over the turkey. Everyone was waiting for dinner, so what could we do? We vacuumed the turkey and served it, telling everyone to eat a lot of mashed potatoes in case we missed a spot. Looking back, we were pretty stupid!

We really loved living at High Point and had no intentions of moving ever again. But, one day I walked into the sales office and told them I heard they were getting good prices for the condos. Was this true? They said, "Can you show it now?" I told them no, my daughter was in the shower. They said they'd give me an hour to get it ready and we got an offer that night that doubled what we paid for it. How could we say No? So we decided to look for a place to move to.

Our Tenth Home

Found a great split level apartment back in Yonkers at a place called Gateway. It was supposed to go co-op in a few months, and we had to buy something within a certain time period because of tax benefits. While we were getting settled, I was notified that my job was ending. The company was in trouble and they had to let me go. So I applied for unemployment while looking for a job. Amy decided she wanted to move to Oregon. She had spent many summers there with brother Joel, Diane and the kids and wanted a new start in life. So we drove her out, left her and our car and flew home. I still remember when Amy came back from her first visit to Oregon. We met her at the airport and she was wearing a cosmic cape and a star on her head. Gerry said, "That's the last time she visits your brother!" He was just kidding, of course. Never saw two brothers-in-law love each other so much.

Still continued camping and Gerry the Cautious One decided to put all of our important papers and cash in the dryer (had a washer/dryer combo, and he figured nobody would ever stand on their toes to find something to steal). Got back from the camping trip and I had a lot of laundry, so I washed away all the remnants of mud and dirt, tossed the clean clothes into the dryer and turned it on. Since it was high up, I couldn't see the "stuff" Gerry hid in it. After about 20 minutes, it dawned on me. We made a dash to the dryer and tall Gerry pulled out all the damp clothes, papers and money. Can't iron wrinkled paper and bills, but at least we didn't set the house on fire! By the way, he never did that again, but still continued to check the doors multiple times before going to sleep. Time passed and the condo still had no signs of going co-op. Our time was running out for the tax break, so we started looking again, and lo and behold, we found a beautiful condo across the Hudson River.

Our Eleventh Home

From Westchester to Rockland County, where I lived as a kid. Did I mention that I moved multiple times until age 10? I was a depression baby and we moved every time my dad got three months free rent. Over the Tappan Zee Bridge to Nanuet, NY to a place called Treetops. It's amazing how we always managed to re-fit our furniture into any area. I used to draw floor plans on a grid and drew furniture to scale. Never threw away the paper furniture because never knew when I'd have to re-figure it. Much easier moving pieces of paper than actual heavy furniture, and it always worked. While living in Treetops, Gerry's assistant at work quit. Since I was still out of work I volunteered to come in and help him for the summer. I was some help! His phone rang one day and I answered it. Caller: Is Gerry there? Me: He's at a meeting. Can I take a message? Caller: Oh, do you work for him? Me: Actually, I sleep with him. Luckily, it didn't cost Gerry his job and I tried to be more discreet. While there, I got bored and offered to do a catalog for the company. Did quite a few, very successfully, and would have liked to work there full time, but they didn't want any husband/wife team on the payroll. Then one day, Gerry got a call from a major lingerie company. They wanted him to come to their company big time. At the interview, they offered him a huge salary increase, a car and full-time employment for me. Gerry went in next day and gave his notice. He loved his job, but this was too good an offer to turn down. Then he got a call from the president of his future company, asking him to meet with their lawyer. Just a formality. Gerry walked into the lawyer's office and had bad vibes. The lawyer said he was going to call the president of Gerry's current company to see if his credentials were legitimate. Gerry offered him names of presidents of some of the largest companies in the garment business that he dealt with. Lawyer still insisted on calling Gerry's boss. Gerry said, "He wants me to stay. What do you think he's going to tell you? There's no way you're calling him." Lawyer persisted. So Gerry told the lawyer to go f*** himself and to keep the job.

We now had a dilemma. Gerry just gave notice to his present company and quit his future company. The president of the company with the lawyer called that night and told him to forget about the lawyer. He wanted him and everything would work out. The next day Gerry spoke to the comptroller of the company he just gave notice to. He said he was having one difficult time making a decision. He really wanted to stay, but the new company offered him so much more... plus the chance to work with his ditsy wife. The comptroller trotted into the office of the prez, and closed the door. I was beyond nervous. Shortly thereafter, Gerry was called into the office of the president (it wasn't even oval). He was told that he would be given a substantial increase, a company car and that they'd hire me full time. And Gerry said, "Let me think about it. I'll let you know tomorrow." WHAT? At this point I couldn't breathe, but Gerry was calm as a cucumber (where did that saying come from?). Next morning, the president ran into our office and Gerry told him he decided to stay. Relief and joy all around. The president from the "lawyer" company continued to call, but Gerry told him to please stop. He was staying with the company he really loved. And we traded our trailer in for a luxury model with a back bedroom and air conditioning. Moved to a nearby camp site called Rayewood, and our whole camping group from Pleasant Acres moved with us: Al and Alice, Bob and Wendy and Carolyn and Rob. Had a big camp fire area that we all shared, and the guitars and folk singing continued way into the night.

FROM PR DIRECTOR TO ART DIRECTOR

Now that I was a real employee, I started doing more
than catalogs Our company screen-printed ladies and
girls sleepwear, and had licenses for Disney, Snoopy,
etc. I thought the garments had very little originality
in the art work, so I started presenting ideas, using
fabric designs in the art (if there was a striped sleeve,
Snoopy would be lying on a matching striped heart).
Before long I was art director for ladies and children
and loved my job! I started traveling to California
for Disney and Snoopy meetings. Sometimes my
boss would look wary when I opened my mouth at
Disney meetings. Can't say that I blamed him. For
instance, at one meeting they were introducing the
Dick Tracy movie which we had to translate into art
work for sleepwear. Then they told us they were doing
a promotion with McDonald's. I blurted out, "Are they
going to have a Mac Dick?" Oops. Luckily, they laughed
and my boss wanted to disappear under the table.
Gerry was vice president in charge of production, and
that meant he had to have the fabric printed in just the
right colors. So I traveled on a regular basis to plants
in North and South Carolina. Printings could last 21
hours straight until they got the color just right. At
first they tried to con me into accepting whatever they
brought out as a sample. If it wasn't what we needed,
they got it right back. I'd tell them what colors to add
or subtract and warned them to use a better pigment or
I'd pull the job. After a while they got the message and
they accepted this Yankee colorist into the fold.

I traveled so much, I didn't have much time to meet our neighbors. One day we looked out at a driveway two doors away, and there was a group of women chatting. Gerry told me to go over and introduce myself, so I took my little folding chair, walked over and settled in for the get-together. They talked about 15 minutes on how to clean a house. I said, "My mother told me not to kill myself so the next one would enjoy it all." One woman said, "I am the next one!" So I took my little folding chair and went back home.

GREAT THINGS HAPPEN

While living at Treetops, Ronni met Mark, they were engaged and got married. My folks were at the wedding and my father got to sing "Always"... same song he sang at our wedding. My mom, Ekka, did her famed belly dance. Amy was living in Oregon, and when told of the wedding wanted to know if it was going to be a real wedding, with soup and everything. Told our friends about her comment, and during the dinner, a whole table of jokesters walked over to Amy's table with their bowls of soup. At the ceremony, the Rabbi called Mark three different names: Mark, Terry, Perry. Mark stepped on the glass three times to make sure he was married. Mark's parents, Fran and Bob, became part of our extended family, as did Lillian, BJ, Freddie and the whole Michelson clan.

Susi was living in New York City and decided to buy a condo in Spring Valley, ten minutes away from us. While there, she was introduced to Matt, our future son-in-law. It was also during this time that we realized we hadn't moved in a while. So we started looking at condos in New Jersey, close to our daughter Ronni, hubby Mark and grandson-soon-to-be-born. Yes, Ronni was expecting. Found a wonderful place called Concordia, off Exit 8A on the NJ Turnpike (in New Jersey, that's how you identify your location). After we bought the condo, we realized we'd have to sell in a hurry. But it was Labor Day weekend, so we went camping. Got home and had camping gear and laundry all over the place, when a broker called and asked if we could show our house. Didn't expect much, so we opened the door, told them to make themselves at home and we kept unpacking. That night we got an offer. It was a little low, so we counter-offered. The next day we got a call at our office. Offer accepted. So we started to pack again, and set the moving date for December 12.

On December 1, 1986, our grandson Eric arrived, weighing in at 10 pounds. In the hospital nursery, he looked like a turkey surrounded by Cornish hens. His delivery was supposed to be at White Plains Hospital, but being from a moving family, Ronni had relocated to Jersey. Her water broke on Thanksgiving Sunday, contractions speeded up on the New Jersey Turnpike Exit 10, and even the police could not get her to White Plains in time. So Eric was born at Hackensack Medical Center. Oh, what a night!

Our Twelfth Home

Moved into Concordia on schedule, Friday, December 12. The movers carried my piano into the living room and said, "Lady, it's not going to fit." I told them I knew it would be fine, because it fit on my graph paper. They thought I was nuts, but accommodated me, and I was right. It fit perfectly. Had no telephone. It was to be installed Monday. And this was the time before cell phones. On Saturday, friends who already lived in Concordia knocked on the door. They had gotten a call from Ronni saying that my father was in the hospital. I went to their house to call Ekka. She said he had a high fever and that one of our friends who lived near her would take her to the hospital to visit him. Nothing we could do at that point, so we returned home, looked at the 86 cartons, and started to unpack.

Joy to Sadness in One Day

Sunday morning, Ronni (the new mommy) rang our
door bell. She came to tell me my father had passed
away. She had a 2-week-old baby and couldn't join us,
but Gerry, Susi, Amy and I drove down for the farewell.
Ekka was not well, and couldn't be left there alone, so
we told her she was coming home with us. Ekka ended
up in the hospital the day of the funeral. I don't think
she could deal with saying goodbye. Susi flew home a
few days later, had to go back to work. Joel helped us
pack up the apartment and then flew back to Oregon.
Gerry and Amy drove back home with a car loaded with
all of Ekka's treasured belongings.

Amy was doing the first lap of the drive when it started
pouring. She hates to drive in the rain, and said,
"Grandpa, give me a rainbow." And the sun came out
and a rainbow appeared directly in front of the car. She
almost ran off the road! Ekka and I flew back a few days
later. An ambulance took her from the hospital to the
airport. We had just moved in, and there were all those
cartons waiting to be unpacked, so Ronni invited Ekka
to stay with her for a few weeks so we could get our
house ready for our new guest.

Ekka enjoyed being with her great grandson so much, and she couldn't wait to tattle on Ronni. Seems the first time Ronni put Eric in the bathtub, she shampooed him, washed him and then drained the tub. Poor soapy baby was sitting in his bathtub seat in an empty tub. Ekka asked what she was doing. Ronni explained that you can't rinse a baby off with dirty water, so she refilled the tub with clean water. She only did this once! New parents always have funny first-time stories.

After two weeks, we moved our bedroom set upstairs, unpacked and bought a bed for Ekka so she could be downstairs in the master suite. We bought a little crib to keep in her bedroom, and Ronni and Eric visited every day while we were at work. Ekka started going downhill very rapidly. She was hospitalized several times, went to a nursing/rehab home for a very short time, and decided she didn't want to hang around without her Irving. She passed away in March of 1987. Within three months I gained a grandson and lost two parents.

In May of 1987, Susi and Matt had a beautiful wedding. Susi and Ronni both wore my original wedding gown (altered, of course). My brother Joel and wife Diane got up to do their very original hippie dance, and we still have photos of Matt's folks, Pat and Marvin, looking a little perplexed. I think Pat was thinking: It's too late. They're already married. The two sides of the family, however, loved each other after officially meeting. Susi and Matt sold their condo in Spring Valley and moved to a beautiful bi-level home in Pine Island, NY… heart of the black dirt region.

Hip Hip Hooray

Gerry had been having hip problems for quite a while, and didn't want to do anything about it until after the wedding. We had to do our famous lindy at Susi's big day. Gerry used to throw me over his knees during this dance. Maybe that's why he had hip problems? In June of 1987, Gerry had his right hip replaced. Surgery was a success and he was a terrific patient. The day he came home from the hospital, his company set up a computer in the house so he could take care of business, and he did it all with his wonderful sense of humor. Being optimists, we always figured that rainbows followed rain.

Went to Florida for the unveiling of Ekka and Irving's gravestones the following year. Amy was still remembering her rainbow gift from Irving. After the ceremony, we all went to the beach, just to look at the ocean and the sky and to feel some peace. Suddenly, across the sky, a double rainbow appeared. From then on, rainbows have always symbolized Ekka and Irving watching over us. When we flew down for the unveiling, we decided that something sad had to turn into something glad, so we bought a condo in Delray Beach, Florida. Since we were still working, we rented it out each year from January through April and spent two weeks of Christmas vacation there. The rent we received paid the mortgage, and we figured we'd have a future home when the time came to retire.

When we bought our Florida condo, we just spent two weeks a year there. Keeping his security mind-set intact, whenever we drove to and from lala land, Gerry would unpack the entire minivan whenever we stopped at a motel. He would also check on the car a few times a night. On our return trip from Florida, he even insisted on bringing the bags of grapefruits into the motel. After we retired and started driving to Colorado for six weeks every summer, I rebelled. Enough with the unpacking every night. My Gerry Boy agreed (reluctantly) and guess what? Nothing was ever taken from the van (but Gerry still looked out of the motel window a few times a night).

After Eric was born, Ronni tried to get in touch with
Evelyn. She thought that after years of discord, Eric
would be the catalyst to bring the family together.
It didn't work. It was so sad. Everyone who ever met
Gerry loved him and respected him... except his
own mother, who was not capable of giving love. For
years we visited Gerry's parents and grandparents
every Sunday, knowing we would be criticized the
minute we walked in the door. We thought it was the
right thing to do, never realizing how much the verbal
abuse was hurting everyone. My loving clan tried to
please a woman who couldn't accept our love, and our
relationship eventually ended.

In September of 1988 Gerry's Uncle Bob passed away,
and Evelyn ended up in the hospital the same day.
Amy called and asked us if she should visit her. We
told her not to go, since she requested that none of her
family be there. We hadn't spoken in many years. Amy
thought maybe she should go to the hospital and peak
in the door. At that time, call waiting beeped, so we
told Amy we'd call her back. The call was from Stanley
saying that Evelyn just died. I called Amy back and told
her, "What we were just talking about, uh, you don't
have to go to the hospital. She just died."

We went to Bob's funeral and Gerry didn't want to add to the family's grief, so we didn't say anything until the family get-together after the service. Bob's wife Irene, who we dearly loved, was Evelyn's sister, and they hadn't spoken in years, either. So we arranged a graveside service the day after Bob's service, and Bob's kids and grandkids all showed up to give Gerry support. It was difficult to mourn someone you lost years ago.

OUR FIRST BOAT

Decided to trade our camping experience for a boating experience. Sold our trailer and bought a 24' Sea Ray. We knew nothing about boating, but always loved the water. We found a marina off Barnegat Bay. After sitting at the dock for a few weeks, waiting for the wind to stop blowing, Gerry finally mustered up the courage to take the boat out. Problem was getting the boat back into the slip. There's no brake (like in a car) and you have to know what you're doing. One day, the guy next to us took his boat out, forgot something and returned to his slip. Captain Gerry paid strict attention and said, "Oh, that's how you do it!" From then on, it was a piece of cake! Of course, the first time he did it the right way, I leaned over the side, grabbed the line to help pull the boat in, and pulled the line in the wrong direction. The boat started leaving the dock. Oops! I did learn to be a pretty good first mate, though.

At the end of summer 1991, we had some very special passengers: Carol and Mike (From the turkey dinner. Mike was now mayor of Ardsley) and Arnold and Harriet (The president of the Rofheart Family Circle). That boat ride stays in my memory, because in a few months they would both pass on. Mike from cancer and Arnold from a massive coronary. How could they leave at such young ages? We were all supposed to retire together.

AND THE GRANDCHILDREN COMETH

When Eric was two years old, Susi gave birth to Nicole, and we delighted in two gorgeous grandkids. A year later, Ronni gave birth to Scott. And the joy continued. Then Andrea arrived in the Wynn household, another beauty, and eventually Ryan would make his way into the Hansen household, a character and a cutie! We felt so blessed. Whoever said, "grandchildren are your dividends" said it right. This paragraph is a little out of order, but I had to set up the wedding that ensues.

Colorado Time

Amy moved out to Colorado in September 1992 and roomed with her girlfriend. Three weeks after the move she went to a roadhouse-type bar named Little Bear and met a guy named Carl. They both went there for the music and ended up together. Four years later, he got up the nerve to propose. They eloped in February of 1996. In the summer of '96 we gave them a "wedding after the wedding." Mark was the "preacher" and after a comedic ceremony, he said to Carl, "I know that you're not Jewish, but since you eat bagels religiously, we're giving you the Hebrew name of BAGELAH." He then presented the couple with a beautifully decorated bagel, which is still gracing their fireplace mantel. Nicole and Andrea were supposed to be flower girls, but Andrea was very young and very shy and backed out at the last minute. Scott said, "Give me the basket," and proceeded to wiggle his tush down the aisle. Still have the picture of Nicole following him and cracking up at the sight.

Our Wonderful Family

Eric (1986) and Scott (1989), sons of Ronni and Mark. Nicole (1988) and Andrea (1992), daughters of Susi and Matt. Ryan (1998), son of Amy and Carl. And what can I say? They are all creative, talented, intelligent, gorgeous, wonderful human beings. Since the grandchildren started speaking, I wrote down all their incredible sayings, dated them and threw the scraps of kid wisdom into a box. Years later I made a book with five chapters, one for each kiddo. They still enjoy reading about what they said way back when. As I write this, Eric has graduated from Rutgers College Business School. What a time to major in finance! Scott is a junior at Rutgers, and is majoring in Criminal Justice. He is also a volunteer fireman in Monmouth Junction, NJ. Nicole is a junior at SUNY Purchase College. She's a graphic design major in their art school, and is on the Dean's list. Andrea is in her junior year at high school and recently performed in a community theater production of Urinetown. Ryan is a sixth grader who loves school and reading and writing short stories. He also loves playing the violin. All of them love music.

Eric and Scott play dueling guitars and get a kick out of playing rap crap when Grammy is a passenger in their car. Ronni and Mark also play guitars and sing the oldies besides writing their own songs. Nicole knows all the pop groups, but still loves Simon and Garfunkel. She wrote a play with their songs threading the way through a very haunting script. Andrea is our singer/dancer. She played a lead role as the baker's wife in Sondheim's "Into the Woods," in her middle school production. Her goal is Broadway. Susi plays guitar and writes and produces amazing school shows. Matt is the expert on every Motown song ever written. Ryan, the Guitar Hero expert, was brought up with music in the house. Amy has had records and then CD's playing daily since he was born. Carl is a very talented composer/musician, and Ryan can be seen playing drums to his daddy's keyboard. I'm not too proud of my kids, am I? One day the grandkids were thinking of names to call us instead of Grandma and Grandpa. Someone suggested Grampy for Gerry and Nicole changed it to Grumpy and that stuck (even though he was anything but grumpy). My name changed to Grammy and I liked that name because it sounded like an award.

OUR SECOND BOAT

Now that we were experienced sailors, we decided that we needed a little more space....especially since the family was growing. Sold the 24' Sea Ray with an 8-foot beam and bought a 28' Sea Ray with a 10-foot beam. First boat was named Hadda Havit. Second one was Hadda Havit II. Spent most weekends rocking in the water and loving every minute. We became personal friends with Sea Tow (I think they moved the buoy markers to get business). Landed on quite a few sand bars, but who cares! We thrived on the water experience. Our kids and grandkids came out as often as possible. Had a great time fishing. I swear the same crab followed our boat every weekend. We'd catch him, throw him back and I think the crab was saying "nah-nah-nah-nah-nah!"

Gerry once got some squid for bait, started to cut it and splat! There was ink all over the boat. He forgot about the "insides." He once caught a fish that I thought was pretty neat, and Captain Gerry said, "Oh, crap. It's a blow fish." Couldn't understand why he was upset. He told me to just watch. All of a sudden the fish blew up into a globe, like a Christmas tree ornament. Threw that back, too. This boat had twin screws (engines, I'm not being rude). Gerry didn't know quite how to handle them. He'd come into the marina too fast, go into reverse too fast, and "tapped" the boat next to us a time or two. Finally, our neighbor decided to let him in on the secret. Turn one engine off and glide in. From then on, Captain Gerry was a pro.

THE SUMMER OF 1995

We came down to the marina with our sons-in-law and loaded the boat with the necessary gear for the season. When Gerry tried to get off the boat, his right leg wouldn't move. The guys helped him off and we went to a local orthopedist who told him the bad news. He needed a right hip revision. He had fallen a few times and the cement they used in the first surgery had cracked, eroding lots of bone. Poor guy was in agony. So the boat sat in the slip — very lonely — and Gerry had the revision done at Robert Woods Johnson Hospital that August. The kids and I went to the marina, unloaded the gear, said good-bye and sold our dream. But, hey, we had other dreams!

We had lived in our New Jersey home for ten years…a record for us! In the Spring of 1997, I was called into my boss's office for my annual review and was told I was no longer needed. Seems everything was going in the direction of computer graphics and I didn't even know what a dot.com was. They gave me a generous goodbye package, including medical coverage until August, when I reached Medicare age. But with basically one income, the time had come to start our move to lala land. Gerry decided to work until August of 1997, so we sold our Jersey home (at a loss) and moved in with Susi temporarily, while getting our Florida home ready. In the Fall of '97, the snowbirds became early birds (that's what they call the people who have dinner at 5 P.M. or earlier to get better prices). Our home was a few blocks away from Gerry's high school chums, Phil and Bev. They are the ones who introduced us to the Palm Greens development.

So We're Retired. What Do We Do Now?

So after working most of our adult lives, here we were
in Florida. We didn't play golf. We didn't play tennis.
We couldn't just sit around and look at palm trees,
so we decided to look for work in the flea markets.
Gerry sold designer sunglasses and eye glasses in one
indoor market, and I sold house wares in another.
There was no pressure, and we loved dealing with
the public. I met some people who looked familiar,
and as we started to talk, we realized we had gone to
school together in Spring Valley... 60 years earlier! I
remember one little old lady asking me the price of
something. When I told her, she said, "Well, maybe I'll
come back tomorrow. I'm a little short today." I said,
"And tomorrow you'll be tall?" Luckily, she laughed!

Cataract Time

In 1999 Gerry went in for cataract surgery on both
eyes, a week apart. This was performed by Dr. Rand
at the Rand Eye Institute. It was quite an experience
as I watched the actual surgery on a TV screen in the
visitors' lounge. Then in 2002 it was my turn. We
always did everything together! My surgery was also
successful. Maybe too successful. When I came home,
the color TV was much brighter. Everything was so
clear and sharp, even the dust on the TV (never noticed
it before). And there were wrinkles under my eyes I
never saw before. That's because my glasses hid them,
and when I took the glasses off I couldn't see them.

DISNEY WORLD

When we moved to Florida, we promised each family a
trip to Disney World. Ronni and Mark were the first to
visit this enchanted place with Eric and Scott. Spent 6
nights at a hotel on the premises and hopped bus rides
to the different areas. The boys were just the right
age to enjoy everything! Actually, Ronni had never
been there either, so she became a kid, even though
she was over forty. Ronni, Gerry and I waved to the 3
boys (Mark became a kid there, too) as they rode the
Water Rides and scary roller coasters. We all went on
the Thunder Mountain ride, and Gerry was taking
movies. When we started taking those dips and turns,
he put the camera on the floor of our car and forgot to
turn it off. All you see are sneakers and all you hear are
screams of joy and fear. We usually kept tabs on
each other by looking for certain clothing colors. Went
to MGM Studios one night and the skies opened up. We
all bought yellow Disney rain slickers. Problem was,
when we left MGM and tried to find each other, there
were hundreds of yellow slickers. Found each other
eventually and had a ball. All the Michelsons loved
the restaurants, and the boys loved the arcades. It was
a magical time in a magical place.

The Wynn turn was next. Matt was not able to get away from work, so he drove Susi and the girls to South Carolina, we drove up from Florida and met at the half way point. Nicole was born with a bone disorder called MHE (multiple hereditary exostoses) and had already gone through a few surgeries. When we went to Mickey land, Nicole was recovering from her latest surgery, so she saw Disney World while zooming around in a wheelchair. One good thing about the wheelchair was it got us ahead of most lines. One bad thing was visiting Norway at Epcot. All the streets were cobblestone and Nicole yelled, "Get me out of here!" She did go on the Thunder Mountain ride once. Wanted to try a roller coaster ride, but it really hurt her "bumpy bones." Andrea loved the cafeteria on the grounds of the hotel, and both girls loved the arcades and gift shops. Those arcades are funny places. You can spend twenty bucks on the games and wind up with a twenty-cent prize and you're thrilled!!!

When Ryan turned five, it was the Hansen turn. Gerry was recovering from a left hip replacement and needed a wheelchair to get around. Again we got to the head of the line, but sometimes Gerry and Carl would go back to the hotel and Amy, Ryan and I would continue the sightseeing. Every time we were about to get on a ride, Ryan decided he had to pee. Finally took him for a pit stop before going on line. He loved the African Safari ride and the train ride around Magic Kingdom. Like his cousins, he loved the arcades!!! And he loved swimming in the hotel pool surrounded by large

Disney characters. Amy and Carl went out one night to Disney Village. We had never ventured there and didn't realize it existed. We all went there one night and had a wonderful dinner. Ryan was very hyper that night and never stopped talking throughout the entire meal. He ate inbetween taking a breath. Very funny night!

BACK TO LALA LAND

It was really beautiful in our Florida home. A canal in our backyard (actually a big puddle) in which ducks and an occasional alligator used to swim. Loved the reflections of the palm trees in the water. We enclosed the back screened porch and made an office/art studio. We enclosed the front screened porch and it became a lanai. In Florida, nobody has a porch! I guess I should mention that it was in Florida that I learned to fill the car with gas. Gerry had surgery on his left hip, and I had to do the honors, since gas stations there don't fill 'er up. He told me explicitly to remove the gas cap, put the nozzle in the tank, do something with the lever at the pump (don't remember if it was up or down) and when the tank was full, to shake the hose like a dick. I followed his directions, and when the tank was full, I removed the hose and started shaking it all over the driveway. He said, "NO! That's not what I meant. Shake it inside the tank so it doesn't leak onto the ground." We loved watching the national weather news when it was freezing up North and we were walking around in shorts. Then medical problems again.

An Unsuspected Diagnosis

In February 2004 I was diagnosed with breast cancer.
Quite a shock! But we found a good surgeon and great
oncologist and scheduled surgery for March 1st. The
surgeon asked if I would be willing to undergo an
experimental procedure called cryosurgery, which
would destroy less good tissue. I agreed, figuring I'd
give it a go if it might help someone else in the future.
After surgery, it was discovered that some cancerous
cells were still present, so on March 15th I had my
second surgery. The sentinel nodes were clean, so I had
a very good recovery chance with chemo and radiation.
Up until this time, Ronni wouldn't fly, but her friend
Ellen said she'd come down with her, and my girl did
what she had to do. Ellen mentioned Ronni's fear of
flying to the flight attendant and the crew gave her
wings (the kind they give kids), knowing she had
overcome her phobia. Ellen returned home after one
week and Ronni stayed till my second surgery and
flew home all by herself. Now she's proud to say she
overcame the phobia, but not the anxiety... but she still
flies. Bravo! So there I was, with one and 3/4 boobs,
concentrating on getting better, when Gerry went in
for a right knee replacement. This was just a few weeks
after my second surgery, but the appointment was
scheduled before my cancer appeared, and we decided
not to postpone it.

Surgery was successful except for one major problem. The surgery left him with a drop foot and nerve damage, and he was in constant pain from that day on. We thought he'd be driving soon, but he could hardly walk. At the same time, I had to start chemo, a half hour away. Because they gave me a "relaxer" with the chemo, I was afraid to drive home alone. Luckily, Rita (a dear friend from way back) volunteered her husband Sy to be my chauffeur for the next few months. Radiation treatments were only ten minutes away, so I drove myself to this place. Interesting machine. Felt like I was lying under a space ship! In July I noticed a strange rash on my left arm. Went to the doctor and discovered that I had shingles. Ugly and painful, but luckily only on the left arm from the shoulder down to the finger tips. Could have been worse. To this day , however, the shingle pain still visits once in a while.

A Phone Call

Susi and Gerry were talking for a few weeks about a suggestion that Susi and Matt had made. They thought it would be a good idea if we left Florida and moved back to New York. Susi has a bi-level house and we could convert the lower level into a wonderful apartment. I told Gerry that I had to concentrate on getting better. I can't think of moving again! Two weeks later, Gerry said that Susi called. I asked him what they were talking about and he said, "What you don't want to talk about." By this time I was through with chemo and radiation treatments and ready for logic and reality. Decided to sell the condo and make

the move. I knew that Mark would take this decision
the hardest. He loved fishing in our backyard and
going to the beach every day. The Michelsons came
down every year. Amy, Carl and Ryan came down
occasionally, and when they couldn't come to us, we
would drive to them. Susi, Matt and the girls came
down before we decided to move in with them. Did a
lot of designing via computer and mail. Susi had to go
through all the mess and noise, but everything was
decided on ahead of time. Sent sketches of bedroom
wall unit, living room bookcases and kitchenette area.
Also turned a half bath into a full one with a large
stall shower. Went to Home Depot and Lowe's and
picked out samples of tile and paint, which the
contractor purchased at their stores nearby. Susi took
care of guiding the whole process and our new home
was finally ready.

Our Fourteenth Home

In March of 2005 we moved up North. Home again.
Best thing we ever did! It was so wonderful being with
our kids and grandkids. We did some remodeling in
the upstairs kitchen and settled in for a wonderful
experience. Gerry and I did the food shopping, I
cooked, Gerry was the salad maker and dishwasher,
and we had a blast. Gerry was also Nicole's chauffeur.
Susi drove her to school every day and the Crumpster

picked her up in the afternoon. We were up
North in time to see Nicole and Scott inducted into
the National Honor Society, graduate from high school
and begin preparations for college. Eric moved into
his upper classman apartment at Rutgers, and we
saw Andrea star in various school shows and ballet
performances. Susi and I even took belly dancing
classes! Life was good.

COLORADO, HERE WE COME

Since Amy moved there, we drove to Colorado every
summer, and stayed for 4-6 weeks after we retired.
Loved spending time with Amy and Carl and getting
re-acquainted with Ryan. Really missed seeing him
grow up! When he was about 4 years old, he was
studying the alphabet in pre-school. The letter that
week was "H," so he brought a toy plastic horse
to school. We picked him up and he told us that
tomorrow he was going to bring a hammer. We were
overjoyed! The kid is a genius! And then he said,
"Maybe I'll also bring a screwdriver." O.K. Genius
came a few years later.

When Ryan was five, he and Amy drove with us to
San Francisco for niece Naomi's wedding. What a fun
time! Stopped at a rest stop in Nevada and there was no
plumbing. Only outhouses. We were petrified. If he fell
in, there was a long drop to the bottom. Amy,

Gerry and I each held a part of him to keep him safe. When Amy asked the caretaker if there was a kid's bathroom, he said, "Lady, I've been here 20 years and we haven't lost a kid yet." But from then on, every time we passed a rest area, Ryan wanted to go pee in a hole. The highlight of his trip.

In 2006 Andrea decided to make the Colorado trip with us...her first time away from home. She was very brave as she waved good bye and cheerful on the first day's trip. Stopped overnight in Ohio, took one look at Andrea and our hearts broke. It dawned on her that she was really away from home and wanted us to turn back. I got into bed with her and we snuggled, but tears were streaming down her cheeks. Gerry, in his infinite wisdom, sat down and told her that it was too far for us to go back and too far for Matt to come and get her, so when we got to Colorado, if she was still homesick, we'd fly her home. She bravely endured the rest of the trip and it turned out to be one of the best summers she ever had. Ryan shared his bedroom with his Cuzzy Buddy. Even though there were bunk beds, no one wanted the top bunk, so Ryan gave Andrea his bed and he slept on the floor. We did a lot of sightseeing and a very special treat was seeing Crosby, Stills, Nash and Young at the Red Rocks Amphitheatre.

Then all of a sudden, Gerry had terrible pain in his legs. Had serious trouble going up the stairs to our bedroom. Andrea's job was to grab him under the arms as he reached the top of the staircase and steady him for his short walk into the bedroom. Went to the doctor, but no one could figure out what was wrong. He still had pain from his drop foot, but this was entirely different.

How Do We Get Home?

Interesting dilemma. We drove to Colorado and now Gerry couldn't drive. He could hardly walk! So we decided that Amy and Ryan would come back with us, and Amy and I would take turns behind the wheel. Amy doesn't like to drive in the rain, and wouldn't you know it! It rained most of the first day, all through Kansas and into Missouri. Finally cleared up and I got a much-needed relief. When we drove into our driveway, Susi came out to greet us and thought Gerry looked like he aged 10 years from the pain. Went to our family doctor who said he thought it may be polymyalgia rheumatica. If it was, the only treatment was prednisone. Well, within two days our Gerry was his old jolly self.

The pain diminished and he felt like a human being again. He felt so good, that we decided to visit Joel and Diane in Mill Valley, CA. When we called to tell our hosts we wanted to visit, Joel asked how long we would be staying. Without hesitation, Gerry said, "We're staying three weeks!" Wow, what chutzpah! But Joel and Diane were very welcoming , and we had such a delightful holiday! Their home is better than a five star hotel, complete with swimming pool, hot tub, sauna and 60 redwood trees on the property. And our nieces, nephews and their kids were all there to add to the enjoyment. Talked about it for weeks, and every time we thought of it, we smiled.

Gerry Boy was feeling so well, that we drove to Orlando, FL in October for the wedding of Susan and Jerry's daughter. Susan is the daughter of our very dear friends, Hannah and Irv, who lived in Yonkers with us and travelled with us on vacations. Hannah used to say that the only time she ever saw a sunset was when we were on vacation. They are both gone over ten years now, and dearly missed. We danced a few slow dances at the wedding, but didn't take a chance on doing our famous lindy.

From there we drove to Palm Harbor to visit cousins Felicia and Marvin. Great visit!! Then drove to Lynchburg, VA to spend time with Stan and Dolores. They knew how much Gerry loved boats, so they made luncheon reservations on a cruise boat that circled Smith Mountain Lake. We got to the boat, boarded, and waited. And waited. And waited. Finally, a loud speaker announced, "We've never done this before, but the weather forecast is so bad, we have to cancel today's trip." Could have left, but we decided to stay on board, have lunch and make believe that we were really cruising. While in Lynchburg, niece Leslie and her hubby Steve treated us to a real southern-style dinner. Drove up to Charlottesville en route home to visit cousin Ruth and dear friend Augie, and got to visit with cousins Alan and Bess. Then we stopped in Maryland overnight to visit cousins Mimi and Danny and their gang of kids and grandkids. It was really amazing, considering Gerry couldn't even walk in August. Had fun with the kids and grandkids during the holidays and everything was looking rosy!

A Hole In The Head

At the end of March 2007, Gerry went for his periodic dermatology appointment. He had a strange growth on his head, and Nicole (in her wisdom) thought he looked like a unicorn. This suspicious growth turned out to be squamous cell cancer. He went to a dermatology surgeon as an outpatient in April. I was in the waiting room, surrounded by patients with bandages in the oddest places: on nose like Bozo the Clown, on arms, on necks, etc., and then out came Gerry with a hole in his head. The cancer was so deep, they had to go all the way down to the bone (in a procedure called Mohs Surgery). So I became Nurse Ratched. Had to cleanse, add meds and bandage twice a day. At first I used bright white bandages and it stood out like a sore thumb. Someone finally mentioned that they make flesh-colored patches, so it wasn't so obvious. One calamity averted. I didn't know it then, but my nursing skills would soon escalate.

Gerry had a terrible chest pain one night. After a few painful episodes, we went to our doctor, who recommended a cardiologist. Results? Heart was in perfect condition. Our doctor then sent us to a gastroenterologist. Figured it was an ulcer. An endoscopy showed something that did not look good, and they sent Gerry for a CAT scan that same day. We were told to come back in two days for a consultation. Friday, April 20, we sat in the office and watched the doctor's face as he said, "This is not what I expected. You have Stage IV esophageal cancer that has metastasized into the lung, stomach and liver. That night, Andrea was starring as the Baker's Wife in Sondheim's "Into the Woods." So we did what any grandparent would do. We went to the show and enjoyed every minute. We also went Saturday night, when Ronni and the gang joined us, and we all denied reality for two wonderful days.

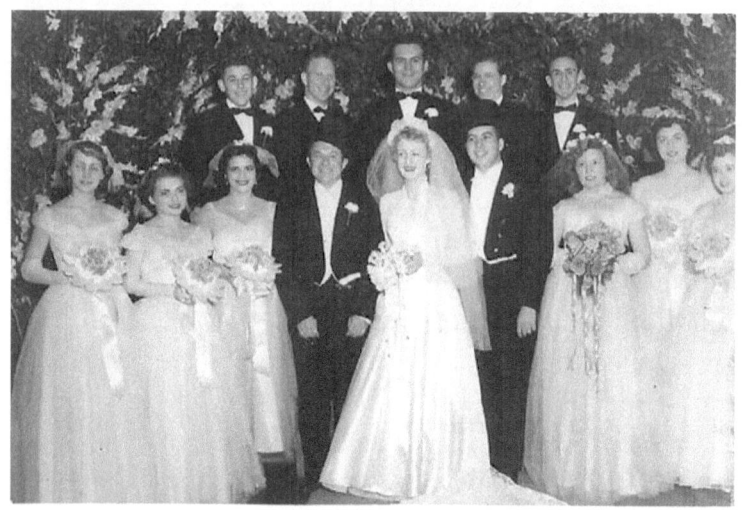

In the beginning there was Audrey, Gerry, and the wedding party.

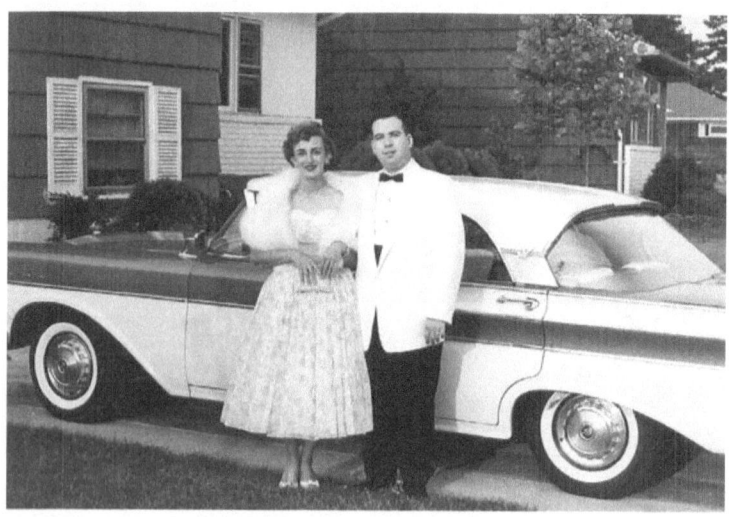

Living it up in East Meadow, NY in the
Fifties.

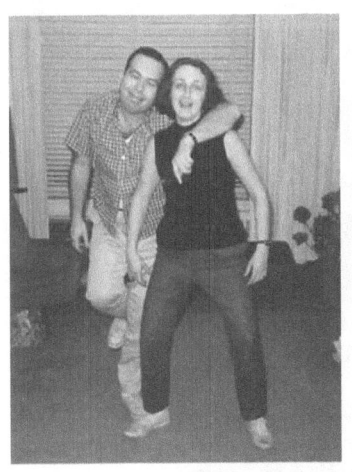

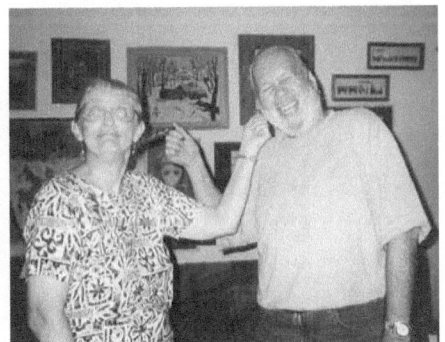

Some things never change...
1971 and 2001.

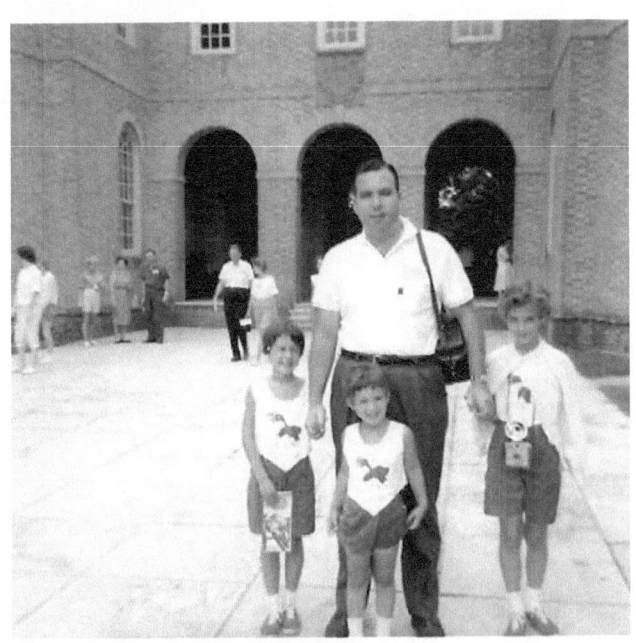

Gerry with his girls (Ronni, Amy, and Susan)
vacationing in Williamsburg, VA, 1959.

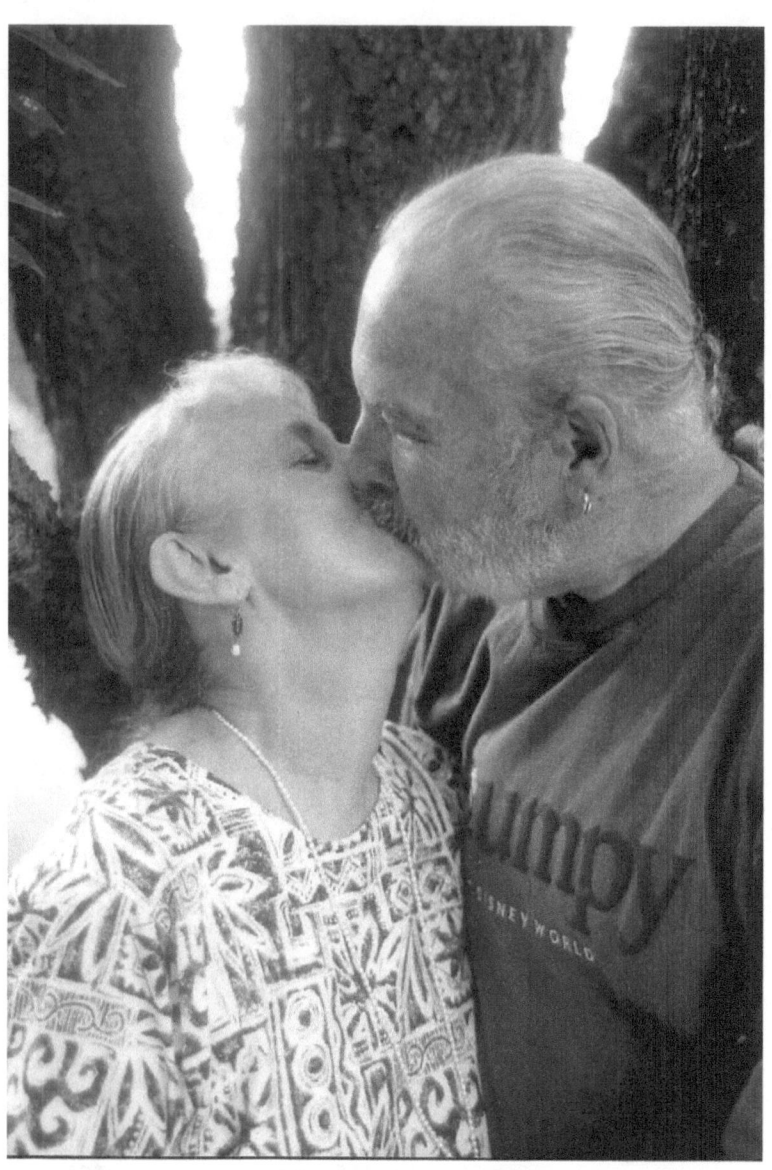

50th anniversary, 2001.

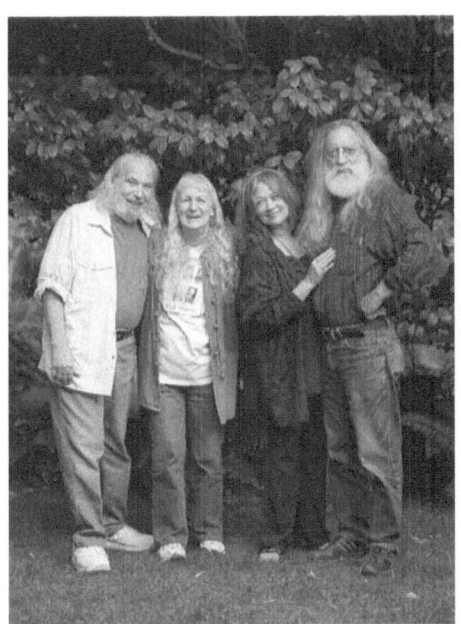

Four hippies in Mill Valley, California.
Gerry, Audrey, Diane, and Joel.

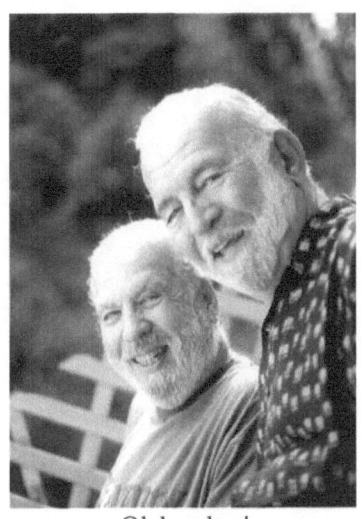

Oh brother!
Gerry and Stanley

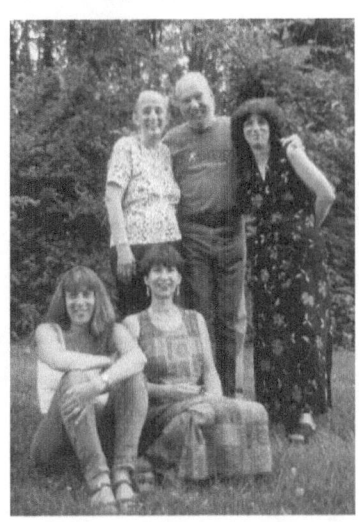

Gerry and his girls at our
50th anniversary party.

Photos by Simeon Schatz

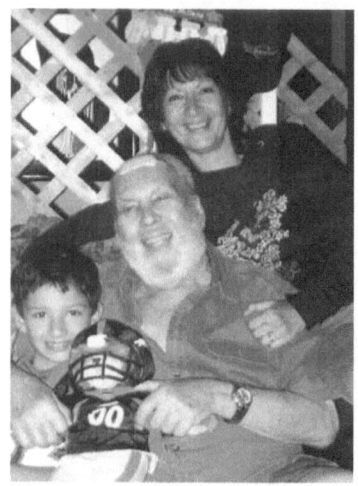

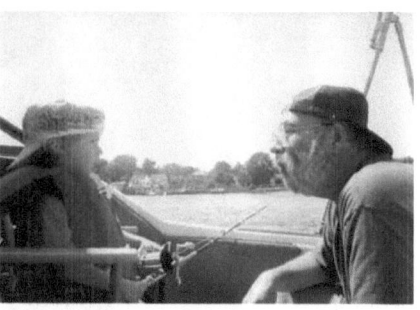

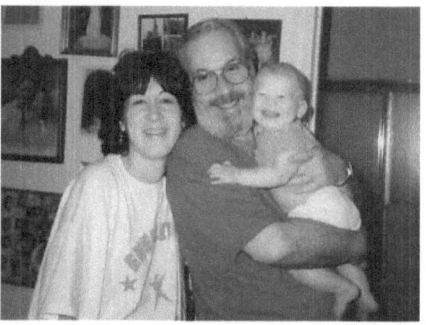

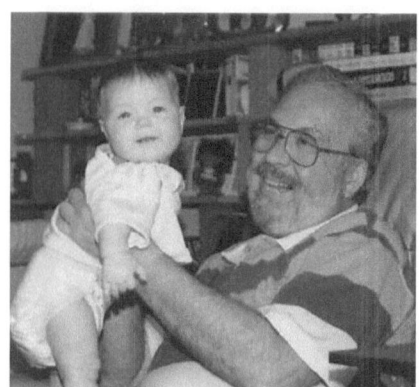

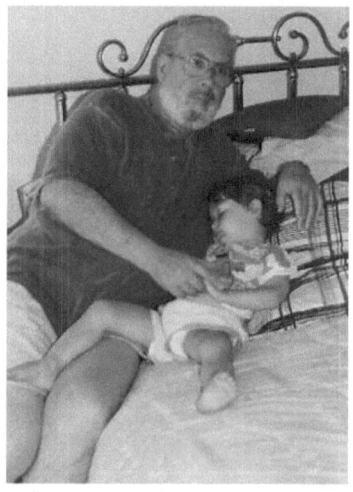

Gerry with the grandkids
(clockwise) Ryan, Scott,
Eric, Andrea, and Nicole.

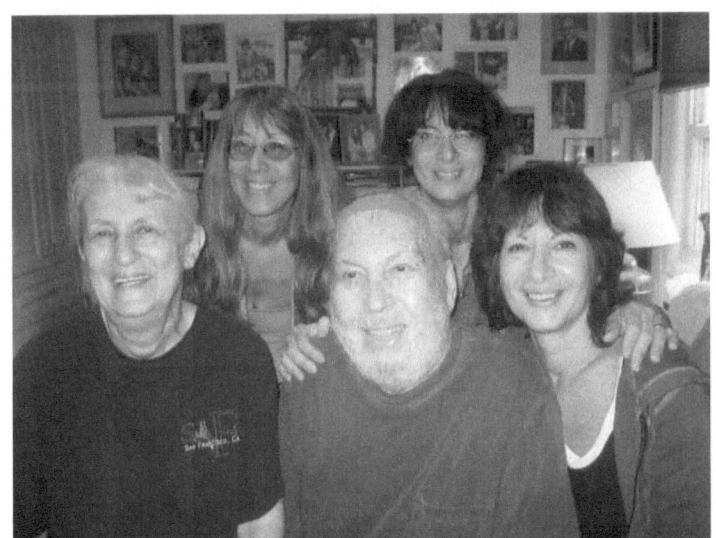

Gerry and his girls (Audrey, Ronni, Susan, Amy), father's day 2007.

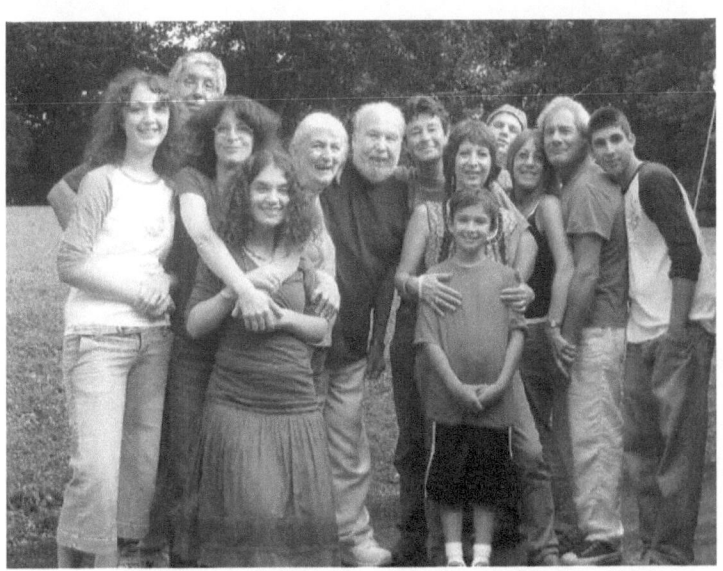

The whole gang at Audrey's 75th "surprise" party, 2007.

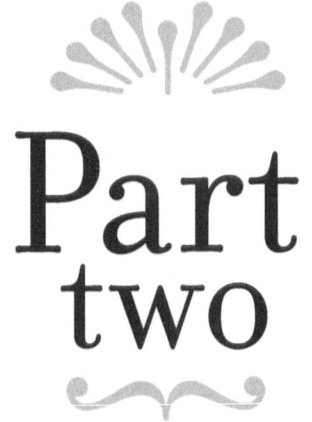

Part
two

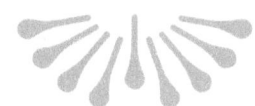

The last 8 months

The Goodbye Journey Begins

Went searching for an oncologist. Our family doctor, Dennis Scharfenberger, recommended Dr. Jane Kanowitz in Middletown, NY, just twenty minutes from our home. We met her, trusted her and knew she was the one. Susi told us of an online site called Caringbridge. org. On April 25 I joined this incredible site, posting daily to let everyone know Gerry's condition. We were supported by thousands of return postings from all over the world. Internet can be wonderful! And cancer became a family affair. Our daughters, sons-in-law and grandchildren were informed of and became part of every decision.

Saturday, April 28, 2007

PET scan today. Other than getting up at 6 A.M., driving 1-1/2 hours to hospital and getting lost in the hospital, it was a piece of cake. Next time we'll drop bread crumbs to find our way back.

Tuesday, May 1, 2007

Gerry had a chemo port and feeding tube inserted today. Port was easy, but feeding tube hurts like hell. Doctor said it would be much better by tomorrow.

WEDNESDAY, MAY 2, 2007

Gerry Boy came home from hospital today. Feeding tube looks like an umbilical cord. Patient wasn't feeling too well today. Pooped out! So we cancelled doctor's appointment and had conference call with her. She said that pet scan was not as alarming as the CAT scan. Sounded encouraging. If he's feeling better tomorrow, he'll start chemo. Susi says he looks like he just had a C-section. He walks like he's doing the C-section shuffle!

THURSDAY, MAY 3, 2007

When I said Gerry was pooped yesterday, that was the wrong expression to use. Shortly thereafter, he had a case of the runs and ran like the Energizer bunny. We'll see Dr. K Monday and start chemo on Tuesday.

SATURDAY, MAY 5, 2007

Grumpy (Gerry's nickname from grandkids) is feeling better today. He decided to get a hair cut and beard trim, and is thrilled that he no longer looks like Einstein. Made a cure-all dinner for tonight. Chicken soup with fluffy matzo balls (Jewish penicillin). He's grinning from ear to ear. Real food! Sure beats Ensure. The chicken soup made him so invigorated, he stayed up till midnight watching "Dream Girls." He was even bopping on the couch!

Sunday, May 6, 2007

O.K. So nobody's perfect. I went to give Gerry 50 cc of water through the feeding tube. Problem is, I poured water in and forgot to release the clamp. Then I took out the "funnel" that holds the water, thinking it had gone down the tube, and the water went all over Grumpy. The bed, the floor, the night table. So he got an unintended bath. Other than that, I've been a good nurse.

Monday, May 7, 2007

Went to Dr. K today (our wonderful oncologist, Jane Kanowitz). Chemo starts tomorrow. She said Gerry will probably lose his hair, but not his beard. Nicole wants to cut off his braid and bronze it! Nice chemo setup. Individual rooms with VHS players. Guess I'll be watching a lot of John Wayne and shoot-em-up movies!

TUESDAY, MAY 8, 2007

Chemo went very well today. We were there over 6 hours. The nurses kept coming in to see if Gerry was O.K., and he was fine. We watched the movie "Score." Our great niece Emma wants to know what chemo is like, so here goes. A tube goes into Gerry's port with assorted liquids dripped in individually from hanging bags. First a saline liquid washes out the system (takes an hour). Then they pour in the chemo chemicals (one at a time) plus anti-nausea meds. At the end, they flush the system again. Since Gerry is a little anemic, he'll get two units of blood tomorrow (through the port) at Tucker Cancer Center in Middletown, NY.

WEDNESDAY, MAY 9, 2007

Went to hospital for blood today. Good vampires. Took 7-1/2 hours, but we had a ball with the other patients. Gerry is now "strong like bull." No reaction to chemo yesterday (knock wood) and he looks and feels great.

THURSDAY, MAY 10, 2007

Went to the "port" doctor today. It took two minutes to remove the steri strips and he said that everything looks great. Gerry is feeling so perky since yesterday's transfusion, he went to Sam's Club and then to Shop Rite. After unpacking all the groceries, he felt a little tired. Doh! When he's not in the mood for eating soft food or drinking Ensure, I pour the Ensure down the feeding tube. Then I pour water down to clean the tube. I'm a nurse in training! My brother Joel suggested that I pour vodka down the tube, but Gerry would rather wait till he can drink it the right way.

FRIDAY, MAY 11, 2007

A quick aside. Our 8-year-old grandson in Colorado brought a Mother's Day card home from school. Proudly, he gave it to our youngest daughter, Amy. It said: "Happy Mother's Day. I'm sorry your daddy has cancer. Love, Ryan."

SATURDAY, MAY 12, 2007

After a relaxing day yesterday (translation: shoot-em-up movies that made me leave the room), Grumpy is planning to join me at Sam's Club. Whoopee! A date! Tonight we go to an elementary school show written and directed by oldest daughter, Susan. Nicole is doing the make-up, Andrea is helping backstage and I wrote a few lyrics. A family affair!

SUNDAY, MAY 13, 2007

Yesterday was not the greatest day for our Gerry. His ankles swelled up from the chemo and the doctor gave him a diuretic. Unfortunately, it worked so well, he couldn't leave the house to go to Susi's show last night. On the bright side, the swelling went down. The show was a smash hit and we're all coming down from that high feeling. Ronni and family visited overnight and Ronni suggested that he cut the diuretic in half. He listened, and had a very comfortable day. Grumpy has been eating soft foods and drinking Ensure, but today he rebelled. He wanted ham and eggs. Grandson Scott cut a small piece of ham into very small pieces. I made very soft scrambled eggs with the ham and he was in heaven! Tonight he was still in the mood for food, so we cut turkey into very small pieces, mixed it with mashed potatoes and smothered it with gravy. What a happy guy!

MONDAY, MAY 14, 2007

Today is the day Gerry and I met... 57 years ago. To celebrate, we went to the surgical supply store for a shower chair and hand-held shower head. We arrived with RX's from the doctor, but Medicare does not pay for safety equipment. They would rather have you fall and break something, and then pay for hospital costs. It figures! Got the stuff anyway, and Gerry can now take a relaxing shower without becoming overtired. Isn't this a romantic way to celebrate 57 years?

Tuesday, May 15, 2007

Grumpy had his second chemo today and he's feeling much stronger. All that liquid and healing stuff dripped into the patient while we watched "The Mask of Zorro." It's like going on a date!

Wednesday, May 16, 2007

When we went to Dr. K yesterday, she discovered that Gerry was dehydrated. That's one of the reasons he's so tired. So it's now 6 cans of Ensure a day plus whatever else he feels like drinking. Don't want to drown the patient! He's doing so much better today, and he's able to drive again. Big help for me. My knee is not doing so well (damn arthritis), and I'm going to rheumatologist tomorrow. This is the way to spend your retirement? The Gerry Boy has a sinus infection that needs antibiotics, Called our family doctor and discovered that he was on vacation until next week. His nurse recommended a Russian doctor in Monroe, NY (30 minutes away) and Gerry said, "Nyet!" I said, "You're going! Can't wait till next week." So off we went and the doctor was wonderful. Turned out he was from Vilna, birthplace of my maternal grandparents . Antibiotics, here we come!!!

Thursday, May 17, 2007

Gerry is feeling better than he did last week. When he doesn't want to drink, I pour Power Ade or Vitamin Water down the tube. I feel like the Statue of Liberty. While the drink is going down and my hand is extended upward, I sing, "Give me your tired, your poor..." (with apologies to Emma Lazarus and Irving Berlin). Poor guy gets nervous. He thinks I'm going to miss, but I can multi-task. Pour and sing at the same time. Now that Gerry can drive, he drove me to rheumatologist today. He shot me in the knee (they shoot horses, don't they?) and ordered a special knee brace that will be ready in about two weeks. This sounds like same brace daughter Amy had before her knee surgery, but I'm not going there.

Friday, May 18, 2007

Went to podiatrist today for regular checkup. Gee, fourth doctor visit this week. Weather has turned chilly-ish (48 degrees), so we'll spend the day inside, Gerry watching shoot-em-up movies and me on the computer.

SATURDAY, MAY 19, 2007

Things have been so great that I almost believed Gerry would by-pass the chemo effects. But unfortunately, the runs started late yesterday. Called doctor, who told me to keep him hydrated. Have been pouring Power Ade down the tube and it's two Immodium every two hours until he feels spunky again. The pooped-out guy (oops, wrong word) is sleeping right now. He was up most of the night, watching basketball reruns at 3 A.M. Immodium finally worked! He's been O.K. since 10 A.M. Have been shoving so much liquid down the tube, Gerry feels like he's treading water. Guess I'll back off. Don't want to become like the real Nurse Ratched.

SUNDAY, MAY 20, 2007

Yesterday was a lost day. Gerry was lying around like a latke (pancake). Maybe I was drowning him. Grumpy realized that when he drank the Power Ade, he was fine. When he got it through the tube, it was not so fine. He's now drinking a lot of Power Ade and has been fine all day. He's even watching movies, basketball and whatever else the remote happens to throw his way. Why can't men watch one thing at a time?

Monday May 21, 2007

We slept almost the whole night. Whoopee! But this morning the runs started again. So we made the trek to Dr. K, who discovered that he was dehydrated again (and I thought I was drowning him). After a few hours of "stuff" through his port, Grumpy was Happy! A new person! So we are home now and Gerry had his first real food in days... a banana! Can't use Ensure for another day or two, but if he keeps on feeling well, I'll make chicken soup with matzo balls tomorrow. And it isn't even a holiday! Can't give the boy what he really wants — a steak. But maybe he'll settle for mashed potatoes and Jello (ugh).

Tuesday May 22, 2007

Went to Dr. K today and visit went well. He's looking and feeling much better than he did a few days ago. Starts chemo again next Wednesday, so we have a little break. Gave the boy two soft-boiled eggs and two pieces of toast with jelly for lunch and he is soooooo happy. Real food!

Wednesday May 23, 2007

Gerry is feeling pretty great today and anxiously awaiting my chicken soup with matzo balls, so I'll cut this short and start cooking.

Thursday May 24, 2007

So far so good. I think the matzo balls did the trick.
In fact, good enough to go shopping at Macy's and
Sam's Club. The Grumpster even had a peanut butter
and jelly sandwich for lunch. Happiness! No plans
for the holiday weekend. Just family, fun, games
and chicken soup.

Friday May 25, 2007

Another great day! Ordered railings to go on our walls
opposite existing railings, so Gerry (and Nicole and me
with the gimpy knee) can hold on both sides for better
balance up and down the stairs. They'll be installed
next week. The patient was getting tired of boiled eggs
and toast, so he had egg in the bread for breakfast.
You know the kind: cut a hole in the center of the
bread, pour in the egg and cook on both sides. Then
he decided that there was something that would make
him even happier. Dunkin' Donuts! So off we went to
indulge our Gerry Boy. Even bought him tuna salad,
which he'll try tomorrow. At this rate, he'll be eating
other foods in no time at all.

Another good day in Pine Island. Daughter Ronni is coming out for a few days...after she sees son Scott dressed in his tux for prom night. Wish I could hide in the bushes to take pix of the cute couple. Scott's prom is another story. The day Gerry was diagnosed with cancer, Scott was in his school parking lot and "bumped" into a car in front of him which hit the car in front of her. So the kids and parents and local police all assembled at the scene where the accident took place. Ronni was speaking to the mother of the girl whose car Scott hit and told her she was waiting for news about Gerry. Everyone at the accident scene was O.K., and that's what matters most. That night, Scott received an e-mail from the girl he hit, wanting to know how his grandpa was. After one or two communications, she asked him if he wanted to go to the prom. What a way to get a prom date! Back to my original thought. Gerry has been very adventurous with food these past few days. From boiled eggs and toast to a slice of pork loin last night, with fettuccini noodles, followed by apple sauce. That is a feast! Getting ready for Amy and Ryan to visit a week from Monday. Grandchildren are even better than chicken soup!

Sunday, May 27, 2007

The adventurous gourmet continues on his quest for real food. Last night he enjoyed tilapia baked in wine sauce and a baked potato. Today for lunch he had a tuna sandwich on a croissant (figured that was soft). After lunch we enjoyed a relaxing movie called "Blood Diamond." Makes you forget any problems you may have, but I can think of more enjoyable ways to spend down time. Great movie, but very intense (thanks for the recommendation, Eric).

Monday, May 28, 2007

After "Blood Diamond" last night, we wanted a light, funny movie, so we watched "Holiday" with Cameron Diaz. Nice change from shoot-em-ups. That didn't last too long, however. I walked into the room where Gerry was watching TV this morning, and it was John Wayne in some war movie, followed by Brando in "Young Lions." That's when I go on the computer. Nurse Ratched hasn'tspilled anything on the patient for a week now. Fast learner. Also found paper tape to keep the long feeding tube in place, so he's very comfortable when I rip it off! Want to share a funny conversation between patient and nurse.
Gerry – You want me to think positive, right?
Me – Right.
Gerry – I want to buy a new grill.
Me – My pleasure (thank goodness he didn't want a new car!).

Tuesday, May 29, 2007

Had our railings installed today. Whoopee! We can all sort of run up and down the stairs without fear of falling. Gerry is really on a roll. His subscription to Yachting Magazine came due for renewal. He said, "I'm renewing it for two years. How's that for positive thinking?" Tonight he will have broiled salmon. Want to give my guy all the good food before chemo starts again.

Wednesday, May 30, 2007

Today was our chemo date again. All 8 hours of it. We watched a movie ("Love of the Game"), had lunch, schmoozed with the nurses, did crosswords and all was great. But, because Gerry's white blood count was a little low, he has to go to Dr. K's office for five days in a row to get a shot of something called Neupogen. Susan and Matt celebrated their 20th anniversary today, and Gerry decided to go grill-looking tomorrow, so we can all celebrate.

Thursday, May 31, 2007

Went to Dr. Kanowitz today. I told her he was there to get shot and she said she hoped he had a bullet-proof vest. After the shot, we went to Home Depot to look for a grill. Saw a really nice one and asked if they could assemble it and deliver it. They said they could do all that, but they would leave it in the driveway. They don't do steps. So we left Home Depot and went to Lowe's. Found a great grill and an umbrella table. They will bring it up to our back porch...all assembled. We expect it sometime next week, and are ready for some serious barbecuing. While we were out, the highlight of the day was lunch. For the first time in a month, we went to a restaurant (Panero's) and had a real lunch date!

FRIDAY, JUNE 1, 2007

Gerry got his second shot today. Everything should be this easy. Stopped at Lowe's again (no more Home Depot) and bought two beer butt chicken holders. Sounds strange, but it makes the most delicious chicken. You put half a can of beer in the holder and put a whole seasoned chicken over it. The poor chicken is standing up and looking so sad, you want to put a dress on it. Sentiment aside, you close the grill and steam it for one to two hours. We'll try it when new grill arrives. Had this delicacy when we visited Amy and Carl last summer. Carl is an excellent cook and introduced us to this dish.

Saturday, June 2, 2007

Today was shot number three. Two to go. Poor guy gets shot every day, but his appetite is still strong. Last night it was chicken livers sautéed in wine sauce with mashed potatoes. His only problem is eating too fast. I tell him to slow it down and eat like I do (but then, he'd never get finished). Ronni dropped by for an overnight visit and we're just chilling today (funny word to use when it's hot and humid).

Sunday June 3, 2007

A funny thing happened on the way home from Gerry's fourth shot. We were obeying the speed limit when a police car pulled us over. O.K. What did we do now? It seems he thought our windows were tinted too dark. Since most cars in state of Florida have dark tints, we did, too. Before we moved back to New York, we asked the tint place to redo the windows to comply with New York standards. Either the standards changed or we were ripped off. Told the officer we were both cancer survivors (don't like the word victim) and really needed the darker tint. He was very sympathetic and gave us a summons (the son of a b****). He told us to get a letter from the doctor and mail it with the summons. That should take care of it. So when Gerry gets his 5th shot tomorrow, we'll get the letter and remain good, law-abiding citizens.

Monday, June 4, 2007

Went to Dr. K today for Gerry's last shot. Asked the office manager for a letter regarding the stupid tinted windows. She never had a request like that before and had to check with the doctor. We went out shopping and by time we called back for the letter, the office was closed. So we'll wait till tomorrow. Amy and Ryan arrive tonight. Yeah!!

Tuesday, June 5, 2007

We are saved! Doctor gave us the letter and hopefully, that's the end of our police saga. Ryan gave Grumpy a Build-A-Bear that he made in Colorado. It has on a Denver Broncos outfit with a t-shirt underneath that says,"Cancer sucks."

Wednesday, June 6, 2007

Long day. Left 9:30 A.M. and returned 5:30 P.M, but chemo went well, and patient is doing well and eating well. Would you believe that after a dinner of linguini and white clam sauce last night, he also had 2 small slices of pepperoni pizza? Way to go, Gerry! By the way, have to thank our long-time friend Carol for the insulated food bag. We bring our lunch in it for every chemo date. Tonight Susi, Amy and I go to an award ceremony at Nicole's high school. She's being given an award for something. Can't wait to find out! Wow! We're back from the award ceremony and our gal received four! Excellence in computer graphics, community service, overcoming hardship to achieve academic excellence and leaders of tomorrow scholarship. So proud of her!

THURSDAY, JUNE 7, 2007

Got a letter from the Town Court today re: the tinted car windows. Our not guilty plea has been accepted and we have to appear in court October 3. I called the dingbats at the court house and said, "If you received the doctor's note and you say the plea is accepted, why do you want him to appear?" They said that you have to hand the doctor's letter to the judge in person. I told them that my husband has cancer, is undergoing chemotherapy and there's no way he can go to court. They said that I could go in his place. I told them that the officer who gave us the summons said the doctor's letter would take care of it. They had deaf ears. I told them to find the officer who ticketed us and let him deliver the letter. Finally, someone offered to walk down the hall and hand said letter to the judge. Doctor's office called today and said they forgot to tell us yesterday that Gerry needs another 5 shots of Neupogen. So he got shot #1 today.

Sweltering day today. In the 90's. Gerry got shot again,
and then we went shopping for steak! You see, new
grill arrived today. The patio table with umbrella
was not delivered, because they couldn't find it. That
will be coming in a few days (I hope), but I still like
dealing with Lowe's. They do steps. Amy's friends from
Junior High, twins Michelle and Monique (who I still
can't tell apart) came out for a quick visit. It's strange
looking at these "kids" and realizing they're
fifty years old! Tonight is Nicole's senior prom. Feel
sorry forthe prom date in his tuxedo in this heat. What
a difference many decades make. Buses pick the kids
up in school parking lot and take them to New York
City... where they board a cruise ship. My prom was in
my high school gym. We decorated with crepe paper
and our parents sat in the bleachers watching us dance.

SATURDAY JUNE 9, 2007

A funny thing happened on the way home from shot
#3. We were following a very slow farm vehicle on a
narrow, no-passing road. Suddenly, a car in back of us
shot out and passed on the solid line and we saw red
lights. The idiot driver never noticed the cop in back of
him. As we passed them, I noticed that it was the same

officer who ticketed us for tinted windows. I wanted to stop and say a few things to him, but Gerry advised me to keep my mouth shut. Ronni and the boys came out today, and Eric and Scott grilled the steak on our brand new barbecue. What a treat! The patient promises to cut the meat into small pieces and eat slowly. Life is good!

SUNDAY, JUNE 10, 2007

Gerry is still smiling about the steak last night. Tonight we'll try turkey with all the fixings. Eric drove back to Jersey, but Scott elected to stay behind to play with his cousin Ryan. Nicole is spending the afternoon with friends and Andrea is baking dozens of cupcakes with decorations for us to consume during Tony Awards tonight. Today was shot #4 and the boy is doing very well. When he's tired, I do the driving, but for the past 2 days he has been boogying down the road! Another of Amy's junior high friends visited today – another Susan. She's been part of our family for years! How can it be that kids get older and we get younger? Tony Awards were fun. Cupcakes were great, and Andrea sang along the whole evening. She probably knows the lyrics to every Broadway show.

Monday, June 11, 2007

Nurse Ratched strikes again! Went to our regular MD because Gerry's blood pressure is a little too low, and his meds need adjusting. Doctor gave him a new blood pressure RX and told him he needs more fluids. When we got home, I figured I'd put some Ensure in his feeding tube for a little pick-me-up. Poured a half bottle into the funnel attached to the tube, turned away for one second and before I knew it, the funnel slipped out of the tube. Ensure was all over Gerry's shirt, the sheets, the night table, the floor, etc. So I cleaned everything up and vowed to be more careful in the future. Good thing I'm not a real nurse!

Tuesday, June 12, 2007

Gerry started running like the Energizer bunny early this morning, but lots of Immodium got him back on track. Went to oncology visit this afternoon, and Dr.K is pleased with his progress so far (especially the eating part). Since he'll probably need the Neupogen shots on a regular basis, and since it's such a shlep every day to get them, we have a plan. If I can get the meds on my insurance plan, they will teach the nurse (moi) and I will shoot Gerry! Amy went with us to the doctor's office and Doc thought she was Ronni. Sometimes those gals look so much alike!

WEDNESDAY, JUNE 13, 2007

Today I had to visit my oncologist in White Plains (follow-up to the breast cancer surgery in 2004). Didn't feel like driving that far, so I called Gerry's doctor and asked if she would mind taking on a new patient. Dr. Jane Kanowitz said she'd love to have me "join the club." Since we do everything together, may as well have the same oncologist. The patient was a little loopy this morning (Ronni would call it disoriented), so I mentioned it to Dr. K's nurse. She assured us it was from the chemo. This afternoon he's back to being our wonderful, nutty Gerry Boy, asking, "What's for dinner?"

THURSDAY, JUNE 14, 2007

Got a call from oncologist's office this morning, telling us that Gerry's potassium count was low. He has to take meds twice a day for three days. So Amy and I did a Sam's Club run and picked up the meds — along with lots of stuff we couldn't resist. Before we left for Sam's Club, I gave the patient a banana. Good nurse, eh? I remembered that bananas were a good potassium source. He's doing much better today. Not loopy. Quiet day today — kids are playing, grown-ups are reading. It's Matt's birthday, but the birthday boy will probably come home his usual 9 P.M. for a late birthday dinner.

I didn't mean to do it. The pharmacist told me to give
Gerry a horse-sized potassium pill yesterday until
she got the powdered ones in. She told me to mash
it and give it to him in water or juice. I thought it
wouldn't taste good, so I opted to give it to him in his
feeding tube. Big mistake! I poured the mixture into
the funnel, unclamped it and it stayed in the funnel.
Oh, oh! I heard that Pepsi clears the tube, so I poured
the potassium mixture back into a glass and filled
the funnel with Pepsi. Unclamped it, and nothing
happened. Now I'm getting nervous. Took a long cotton
swab stick and inserted the wood side into the tube.
After a half an hour of panic, the tube opened up. We're
back in business. Since he started on the potassium
and bananas, he's feeling much better. Yeah! Thought
I'd mention a cute comment from Ryan last night. I
was watching Tiger Woods on the news and the 8-year-
old said, "He's the man behind the legend. I just don't
know who the legend is."

SATURDAY, JUNE 16, 2007

Ironic happenings. Doc gave Gerry potassium because the "runs" depleted it. He was feeling fine until he started taking potassium, and guess what? It gave him the runs. One more day of the potassium cure. At least the powdered stuff dissolves in the water and goes right down the tube!!! Ronni, Mark and the boys came out today. Full house except for Carl, visiting his family in Michigan. We realized that Grumpy would feel very comfortable with drawstring sweat pants, so Mark, Ronni and I went to Macy's . Mark flies through the store and you have to run to keep up with him, but they gave him a great sweat suit for Father's Day. Patient went for a hair cut and beard trim today, so he's feeling mighty perky!

SUNDAY, JUNE 17, 2007

What a great day! Celebrated Father's Day, Nicole and Scott graduating from high school, Andrea graduating from middle school, Eric moving up to senior year at Rutgers and Ryan moving up to 4th grade. Also celebrated Susan and Matt's birthdays and Ronni and Mark's anniversary. Since Ryan will turn nine next month in Colorado, we had a mini pre-birthday party, and best of all: Gerry ate a small rib eye steak – plus zucchini and potatoes from the grill. A super day!

MONDAY, JUNE 18, 2007

Gerry made a few trips to the john in the middle of
the night (thank you, lasix). He started getting very
dizzy and the room was spinning all around. He
remembered that 15 years ago, he had vertigo (no
relation to Hitchcock movie with Jimmy Stewart).
Spoke to the doc, and it's the medicine that's making
him loopy. Yesterday was super for him. Today was not
so super. Here's to a better tomorrow. Amy and Ryan
left at 6 A.M. this morning. We ordered a car to take
them to the airport and it turned out to be a stretch
limo. Ryan was in heaven! When they arrived in
Denver, Amy called to say "The eagle has landed." Miss
those guys, but they're coming back in August.

TUESDAY, JUNE 19, 2007

He's back! Loopy Gerry from yesterday has
disappeared and the patient was chipper enough to go
to chemo today. That Meclizine is a miracle pill. And,
Nurse Ratched gave him a Procrit shot at
the doctor's office. Piece of cake! Waiting for the
Neupogen meds to arrive, so we'll have to make the
trek to the doctor's office for a few more days.

WEDNESDAY, JUNE 20, 2007

Between today and two days ago, we are looking at a new and revitalized man. Went to doc's office for his Neupogen shot. They'll shoot again tomorrow and then it's my turn (if meds arrive). The boy who had no appetite for days is now asking for all kinds of food. In fact, he went grocery shopping with Susi today and they came back with lots of goodies. I even made him a shake that Amy's hubby Carl invented. Root beer, chocolate ice cream and a banana in the blender. By the way, I was giving Grumpy water through the feeding tube, and as I poured it into the funnel, he coughed. The water fountain/spout was NOT my fault!

THURSDAY, JUNE 21, 2007

Went to doc's office for Gerry's Neupogen shot, and guess what? I shot him! Getting pretty good at this nursing business. After doctor's visit, we went to Sam's Club pharmacy and hallelujah! The meds were there! No more driving every day for something we can do at home. Boy is still eating up a storm… in small quantities. But we're thrilled that he's able to swallow everything. Ronni and Mark brought spare ribs from a favorite restaurant, and Gerry's devouring them! Tonight Susi is preparing chili, another favorite dish. Today was Andrea's last day of middle school. Since Nicole will be off to college, they switched bedrooms so Andrea could have the larger room. Always something going on in this household and I love it!!!

Very interesting day. First of all, I shot Gerry and did a
very professional job. Had an uneventful day until the
patio table and umbrella arrived. Andrea announced
that the Lowe's truck was pulling into the driveway. I
ran outside to meet them. Gerry got up from his chair
way too fast, walked toward the garage and slipped slow
motion to the floor (a la Arte Johnson on Laugh-In).
Vertigo has not completely disappeared and the patient
can't do any more get-up-fast tricks. Aside from a cut
on his leg and arm, he's in fine shape. The delivery
men were wonderful. They waited until he wasn't dizzy
any more, lifted him up and walked him to his bed. We
wanted to give them some money, but they refused. All
they wanted was a handshake from the patient. Told
you we loved Lowe's.

Better day today than yesterday. Gerry didn't fall down
once! His leg was "leaking" though. When he fell, he
opened up his swollen leg and I guess the water he was
retaining found a new path to exit. Nurse Ratched is
doing a good job patching up the Gerry Boy. Gave him
his shot again this morning and it was so easy! He's
really not up to sitting on football stadium bleachers
for hours, so Ronni came out to keep Gerry company
and I'll go to Nicole's graduation with the Wynn
family tonight. Sherry and Jim came out to spend the
afternoon with us. Three to three and a half hours
each way. That's pure love. Graduation night was

wonderful. About 400 kids (and Nicole was #32 in the class standings). Being that her last name is Wynn, we had to wait for 390 kids to receive their diplomas. Matt borrowed a bull horn from another parent and we made a ruckus when her name was announced. In fact, we made such a ruckus, we didn't hear them announce that Nicole won another award from the Warwick Lions Club for Community Service. We had a wonderful evening, and Ronni had a wonderful evening with her "poppy."

SUNDAY, JUNE 24, 2007

This morning the vertigo kid was still a little dizzy, but he was revitalized by a phone call from his cousin Alvin (from Florida). Alvin was in Jersey and wanted to stop by on his way back to lala land. Was going to give him directions, but he said, "Don't need them. I'll see you in 2 hours." And he arrived in exactly 2 hours. Drove through the boondocks via GPS. Technology is amazing!

MONDAY, JUNE 25, 2007

The vertigo kid is doing better than yesterday. However, he still gets dizzy when walking. Susi found a walker in the garage and he was using it last night and this morning. In fact, we took it to his GP visit, so he didn't have to worry about falling. Noticed that he looked a little strange walking with it. Turns out it was Nicole's walker, and he was stooping over to reach the handles. When we returned from doctor's visit, Susi found Gerry's walker (about 8 inches higher than Nicole's) and he can now straighten up and fly right (or walk right). Tomorrow is chemo day, so we'd better get books and movies ready for our "date."

TUESDAY, JUNE 26, 2007

Gerry had good chemo session today. When they checked his blood, it turned out that he's very anemic (thanks, chemo). So tomorrow we spend about 6 hours together while he gets a transfusion. We scheduled his CAT scan for Thursday, and so we should have good results by next week. Tomorrow we start the Neupogen shots again. I'm such a pro, I should be wearing a nurse's cap. Hopefully, the transfusion will make him peppy!

WEDNESDAY, JUNE 27, 2007

Just got back from 7 hours at Tucker Center in Middletown where Gerry Boy got 2 units of blood. He's feeling much better than yesterday. I shoot him in the morning for the white count and they drip the vampire stuff all day for the red count. Pretty neat! Between 6 hours yesterday and 7 hours today, I finished two James Patterson books. Relaxing now and getting ready for CAT scan tomorrow.

Thursday, June 28, 2007

Gerry is doing much better today. In fact, he graduated from walker to cane. Today was CAT scan day. We got there on time and the nurse said, "Did you drink the two drinks?" What two drinks? Oops. The receptionist forgot to tell us to pick up the gook and drink it 1-1/2 hours before the procedure. So he drank it there, and we waited 1-1/2 hours for the five-minute scan. This evening we got a call from Dr. K. She called to say she heard from the radiologist, and the cancer had shrunk considerably. I asked her if it was just in the esophagus, and she said no…all the cancers, all over his body. He seems to have some sort of pulmonary infection, though, and is now on antibiotics until he sees a pulmonary doctor on Tuesday. But, hey, we heard good news for a change. My kids always kid me about writing everything with rose-colored glasses. I have to think positive. That's how I deal with disaster. Their friends read my comments on Caring Bridge site and call them up saying, "How is he? Really!" As of this day, my Gerry Boy is great!

Friday, June 29, 2007

Still grinning over yesterday's news. Seems surreal. We just keep hoping for good news at each milestone. Gerry was tired this morning. Aftermath of the CAT scan and drinking that gook. But this afternoon he's back to being his old darling self. In fact, he isn't even using a cane!

Saturday, June 30, 2007

Quiet day today. No doctors, no tests, no shopping. Yeah!!! Gave the patient his shot this morning and I am getting so good, don't even need a band-aid afterwards. This afternoon Susi talked Gerry into going outside for a while. They sat on comfy chairs in the driveway for an hour and a half while the nurse relaxed with a new book. Days like this don't come by too often.

Sunday, July 1, 2007

Four or five days after second chemo treatment, Gerry usually starts "running." This time was no exception. At 3 A.M. the runs started (isn't anything sacred?). By 10 A.M. the Immodium started to work. So far so good. Plenty of toast and jelly, bananas and Gatorade on the menu, and he's starting to feel pretty good right now. In fact, we just finished watching "The Last of the Mohicans." Beats John Wayne!

Monday, July 2, 2007

Today was dentist day for Susi, Nicole, Andrea and yours truly. Since we love our Neal in Somerville, NJ, we made the 1-1/2 hour trek and spent most of the day there. Ronni made the reverse trip from Jersey this morning, arriving at 7:30 A.M. to keep Grumpy company for the day. He spent time on the deck, under the new umbrella, while Ronni played guitar and serenaded him with his favorite folk songs. Not too shabby, eh? Tomorrow is oncology/pulmonary day.

A long day. We left at 10:45 A.M. and arrived home at
6:45 P.M. Sort of a comedy of errors. They changed
Gerry's oncology appointment time, but forgot to tell
us. Waited an hour for his visit. Then we had to wait
another 1-1/2 hours for my appointment, since this
was my first visit since I changed oncologists. Both
visits were fine, but since Gerry had a lot of swelling
on his leg, Dr. K suspected a blood clot. Off we went to
the hospital for a Doppler X-ray, and sure enough — a
clot appeared below his left knee. Have to go back next
week for another picture so they can do a comparison
of the two. If clot stays same size, we do nothing. If it
grows, we do something…like going to the hospital
and getting a filter installed. This prevents clot
from moving to dangerous areas. Next — we went to
pulmonary doctor. It seems that when Gerry's problem
first started and he had trouble swallowing, some
food lodged in the lung instead of in the esophagus. It
became infected and there are pockets in the lung
that must be treated with antibiotics for 6 weeks.
Good news is no chemo while he's on antibiotics.
Bad news is no chemo while on antibiotics. Susi and
Ronni joined us on today's expedition, and Gerry is
looking forward to a break in the routine. What a way
to spend family time!

Wednesday, July 4, 2007

Compared to yesterday, today was wonderful! Just relaxing on this Independence Day. Luckily, I have a good pill cutter. The antibiotics are horse-sized, so I cut away and make them swallowable (Is that a word?). Nicole cleaned up her wheelchair in case Grumpy wants to go outside and may still feel dizzy. We ordered foam pillows and neck pillows that arrived yesterday. Soooo comfortable! If anyone has a neck problem, we highly recommend them.

Thursday, July 5, 2007

Set the alarm for 8 A.M., turned it off and went back to sleep. We were awakened at 8:30 A.M. by Dr. K's office, telling us that Gerry's potassium was low. So I'm dumping potassium down the tube twice a day for four days (doesn't sound very professional, should have said "pouring" it down). After first dose he already started to perk up. Susi and Grumpy watched an episode of "The Shield" this afternoon. Think I'd rather be watching HGTV decorating shows!

Friday, July 6, 2007

What a difference a day makes. Since the Grumpster has been getting potassium, he is a different person. Looks better, feels better and is his old smiling self again. Nicole went for her driving test today and she passed with 100% score. What a happy girl! Susi went shopping for tomorrow's barbecue, when the Michelson clan comes out. She's really a good sport. Since moving into farm country, with little lambs across the street, she stopped eating lamb chops. Didn't want to eat her neighbors. But Gerry has been yearning for them, so she is buying the forbidden meat for us and Matt and everyone else without a conscience!

Saturday, July 7, 2007

What a happy guy is our Gerry! He had lamb chops from his new grill! Actually, he had one chop and four bones from all of us who didn't want dirty fingers. The Michelson men did the grilling, Andrea made the salad, Nicole set the table, Susi made the veggies, Ronni did the dishes… and Gerry and I did nothing but eat and enjoy ourselves. Matt had to work today, but he has a feast waiting for him when he comes home. Gerry is still doing well, thanks to the potassium, and the company helps you to concentrate on fun stuff instead of health issues.

Sunday, July 8, 2007

Another good day. Started by watching Wimbledon
tennis with Ronni and Mark. Incredible match. I
love to watch people do what I can't. Today is the last
potassium day. Hope the pepped-up boy continues
to feel stronger. Tonight he gets more lamb chops.
Susi put some away for him before they were all
devoured by hungry boys (Eric and Scott eat and eat
and eat…). And we hear our Andrea upstairs singing
and singing and singing…).

Monday, July 9, 2007

Our Ryan is 9 years old today. Went for the Doppler
test to see if blood clot had diminished. For the first
time in a long time, Gerry had very little swelling and
very little water in the leg. It even felt good to walk,
so we were unpleasantly surprised when the doctor
told us the clot got a little larger. Next step is filter
insertion which will prevent the clot from moving to
the lung. They assured Gerry that he would be in lala
land during the procedure. Too bad they don't give the
"nurse" some lala goodies while she's waiting.

Tuesday, July 10, 2007

Procedure was scheduled for 10:30 A.M. Due to several emergencies, they brought Gerry into surgery at 3 P.M. But all's well that ends well (according to some famous poet dude named Will). He now has a fancy "umbrella" inserted to catch any clots that decide to wander. Couldn't eat or drink 4 hours prior to surgery, which means his last drink was 6:30 A.M. He finally had something to eat at 4:30 P.M. and that Gerry Boy is one hungry guy! He's resting comfortably now and watching shoot-em-up movies. An aside: On the way to surgery this afternoon, he said, "I remember that we bought bacon last week. I want bacon and eggs for breakfast tomorrow." Guess the vision of breakfast made the procedure a snap!

Wednesday, July 11, 2007

After the long day yesterday, we slept until 10 A.M. this morning, so breakfast turned into brunch. Susi served us downstairs and Gerry had his bacon and eggs with rye toast. I had mini waffles and bacon. A few hours later Susi asked if we wanted lunch. I wasn't hungry at all, but Gerry said, "SURE!" He had a grilled Jarlsberg cheese and tomato sandwich, and ate it in two minutes flat. Since he stopped chemo for a few weeks, his taste buds have changed and he's enjoying food again.

Another strange thing happened. The swelling in his leg went down two days ago and has not returned. Can't figure out where the water went. Our great nephew Jackson would have an answer to that one. "He dwipping pee pee." Now that Gerry is on a food roll, we spent the afternoon watching the Top Chef Marathon.

THURSDAY, JULY 12, 2007

Yesterday's rain dropped the hot temperatures, so we can breathe outdoors again. It was so nice today, Gerry and I took a drive. Not only that, but Gerry drove! When we told Amy that we went out for a drive she was ecstatic…until we told her the destination of our drive. We drove to a local funeral home to make final prepaid arrangements for both of us (why bother the kids when the time comes?). While we were out, Susi, Nicole and Andrea had a painting project. They repainted Andrea's bedroom. Since the girls switched rooms, they each wanted to redo the décor. Methinks they're watching too many decorating shows. Andrea's room is beautiful and Nicole painted a huge "sun" headboard on the wall. We're feeling a lot more comfortable now that the patient has that filter inserted. Now we have to see how long it takes for the lung infection to clear so he can start chemo again. We haven't been able to venture far from home…not even to Ronni, who lives two hours away. Taking everything a day at a time. Now it's time for the nurse to become the chef. The hungry man has requested broiled salmon for dinner.

FRIDAY, JULY 13, 2007

Strange day today. Waiting for rain to arrive and we're all achy. Grumpy had enough meandering yesterday and decided to stay put today. My knee went out this morning, so I'm wearing the brace I got a while back. It's the mother of all braces and seems to help. Nicole has a couple of nerves that are "caught" in her bumpy bones, so she wrapped them and continues with her project for the day: decoupaging a cane/chair. Susi and Andrea did the week's shopping and are both pooped out. I was thinking of going to a movie with Gerry, but just found out that the theater was flooded out last night when a sprinkler system in the floor above broke and poured down into the theater. This was Harry Potter opening weekend. Come to think of it, with the scar on his forehead from the skin cancer surgery, Gerry looks like Harry Potter!

SATURDAY, JULY 14, 2007

What a beautiful day today. The patient and the nurse sat outside for 2-1/2 hours, reading. And then Ronni drove up for an overnight visit. Always a pick-me-up! Susi, Nicole and Andrea went into town for haircuts. When I say town, it's an exaggeration. Town is a deli, a liquor store, a beauty parlor, a farmer's market and two gas stations. But we love this country living. Gerry is having a good day, and as Andrea said, "Grumpy is back!"

SUNDAY, JULY 15, 2007

Sunny day, but too hot for Gerry to sit outside, so he and Ronni visited while Susi, Nicole, Andrea and I went to Warwick for the annual sidewalk sale. Love this funky town with its funky shops. Patient is doing well, feeling well and eating well. Tomorrow is the oncologist. Tuesday, the pulmonary man!

MONDAY, JULY 16, 2007

Went to Dr. K today and Gerry drove. Yeah! He's doing well, but is still a little anemic. So Thursday he gets another transfusion. Today Nicole, Susi and Matt went to SUNY Purchase for Nicole's college orientation. They stay overnight, so we have Andrea all to ourselves. Right now she is reading "To Kill a Mockingbird." I once wanted to name a drink Tequila Mockingbird, but no one took me seriously.

TUESDAY, JULY 17, 2007

Pulmonary doctor today. Hole-in-the-head doctor is tomorrow (to remove stitches from Mohs surgery in April). Today's report was a good one. X-ray taken before the appointment showed that lung infection is almost gone. He has to keep taking antibiotics for another 3 weeks, but can start chemo whenever oncologist thinks it's appropriate. Nicole had a great time at orientation, as did her mom and dad. Don't have to pass the Kleenex until the day she actually leaves for college.

WEDNESDAY, JULY 18, 2007

Went to dermatologist and the wound from skin cancer has healed, stitches have been removed, and aside from the Harry Potter scar, subject is closed. No more cleaning, antibioticing and bandaging. From there we went to hospital to get Gerry's blood cross-checked for tomorrow's transfusion. What a way to spend your retirement!

THURSDAY, JULY 19, 2007

Today was vampire day. Two units of blood and seven hours later we were on the way home. What a romantic "date." Read a new James Patterson book, had lunch and schmoozed with the nurses. It poured all day and I got a little worried, because I left the umbrellas in the car. Duh! But 15 minutes before we left the hospital, the sun came out. This weekend Susi is hosting her annual MHE Gathering. Can't wait to meet all the new and old members with bumpy bones.

FRIDAY JULY 20, 2007

Today the patient tried some exercises on his stationary bike. Took a while to get on the seat since his left leg doesn't want to leave the ground. But he got up there with a little "goose" from the nurse and did 6 minutes. Easier getting off. Just slid off the back! Then we did a couple of laps around the super market. Enough for one day. Have to save our energy for the MHE gathering tomorrow. Our first guest, Anita, arrived from Canada.She'll be bunking with Nicole for a few days. Just spoke to my niece Naomi in San Francisco to see how the family fared during the earthquake today. All O.K. Groceries fell off the shelves in the stores and a few things fell off the shelves in their house, but at least Cameron didn't fall off the top of his bunk bed.

SATURDAY, JULY 21, 2007

A beautiful day for our MHE Gathering. Had folks here from New York, New Jersey, Pennsylvania and Canada. It was wonderful meeting the DeBlasio family, who have been writing on Grumpy's Caring Bridge site, and calling him to lift his spirits. Folks who couldn't make the trip called in from Wisconsin, Ohio and Connecticut. The patient had a great time with all the company, and he looked great without the bandage on his forehead. After the gathering, our ritual has been to take a group photo. Gerry walked out the front door, went to step down onto the grass and lost his footing. Down he went. Scared the hell out of everybody! When he got into a sitting position, Ronni sat down next to him and beckoned the group over. So we all gathered around, kneeling down and we took our group picture with Gerry beaming like a hunk o' hunk as the ladies all had their arms around him. The young man who Nicole went to the prom with arrived bearing graduation gifts. He thought it was a graduation party, so the two recent graduates donned their caps and gowns and posed for pictures. Quite a remarkable day when "bumpy bone" people get together!

SUNDAY, JULY 22, 2007

Ronni and Scott came out yesterday to help with the gathering and they left today, taking Susi with them. She has a very long dental appointment tomorrow with Dr. Neal and Ronni is only 20 minutes away from his office. Ronni will drop her off before she goes to work. Susi is bringing the new Harry Potter, and she'll get lost in Muggleland until Ronni picks her up. Matt will detour to Jersey on the way home from work and we'll see them later tomorrow night. Gerry is having a good day today, resting after all the company yesterday. And Amy, who bought Harry Potter yesterday, is filling Andrea in on all the details via phone. Andrea couldn't wait to find out who bites the dust.

MONDAY, JULY 23, 2007

Today was oncology day, and Gerry told Dr. K that he felt a little funny this week when he swallowed. Felt almost the same as he did before he started chemo. Guess the cancer decided to rear its ugly head again after four weeks of antibiotics and no chemo. So tomorrow he starts again! Anita left for Canada today and the house is getting back to normal...although "normal" is a relative word. We're finding it normal to deal with the ups and downs of cancer.

Tuesday, July 24, 2007

Just got back from our chemo date. The patient did great, and guess what? I get to shoot him starting tomorrow...for five days straight. Even though his white blood count was good yesterday, it will go down after today's session. When we came home, a surprise awaited us. Susi and the girls cleaned our whole apartment. Now we don't have to take allergy pills!

Wednesday, July 25, 2007

Today I gave Gerry his first Neupogen shot. It's been a while, but I didn't forget how to do it. Then we went to rheumatologist and the "shooter" got shot. Got a cortisone injection in the bum knee and I feel much better!

Thursday, July 26, 2007

Patient is doing very well. Went shopping with me in the morning and with Susi in the afternoon. When we went to rheumatologist yesterday, he suggested that Gerry should go to physical therapy to build up his arm and leg muscles. We stopped into PT and they don't have any openings for an evaluation until August 9, so he will ride the stationary bike and lift 2 or 3 pound weights until then.

Friday, July 27, 2007

The boy is looking good today. Guess those shots are working. We went for our regular visit to our podiatrist this morning (for our Medicare Pedicure). Then our niece Sherry and nephew Jim drove up from South Jersey for lunch and a killer game of dominoes. Enjoying the good times for as long as they last.

Saturday, July 28, 2007

Today is a lazy day. Susi is still reading Harry Potter. She did not look at the back of the book first to see the ending, so we'll be quiet and not disclose what Amy told us. Gerry and I watched "Letters From Iwo Jima." Quite an intense movie! Amy called from Colorado to say they all saw "The Simpsons Movie" and loved it! Nicole and Andrea are resting up for trip to Mall tomorrow for school clothes. Ronni and Mark took Scott shopping today for college stuff. Boy, I remember those days!

Sunday, July 29, 2007

Another relaxing day. Gerry is using the exercise bike. Trying to get some strength back in his arms and legs. The Wynns left early this morning for a trip to a very large mall in West Nyack (complete with merry-go-round). Can't wait for the fashion show when they return. If all goes well, we may try to go to our first movie in months (The Simpsons Movie). Since Tuesday is chemo again, it's the only chance we'll have for a while.

Monday, July 30, 2007

Gerry was a little timid about sitting in the movies
for two hours, so he stayed home with Susi and I took
Nicole and Andrea to see "The Simpsons Movie". Such
fun! Last night was the fashion show from the girls'
shopping trip and tomorrow is chemo, so we're getting
books ready for our "date."

Tuesday, July 31, 2007

Our chemo date went well. We both read our books,
ate our lunch and kibbitzed with the nurses and
doctor...all while the healing poison dripped into the
patient. Next week we go just for blood test. I get to
shoot Gerry with Neupogen for next 5 days, starting
tomorrow. August 14 is next chemo date, and then he
gets a little break for a week or so. Want him to feel
good for my 75th Birthday at the end of August. A few
close relatives and friends and neighbors are coming
for my "surprise" party. Correction. Semi-surprise
party. I gave them the list of guests and now it's in their
capable hands. Just love the whispering and funny
looks going around!

Wednesday, August 1, 2007

Got a call from Dr. K's office today. Gerry's potassium
level is low, but we're experts now. Will mix potassium
powder with water and pour it down his tube. Other
than that, the boy is doing well. Even drove to the super
market today and went shopping with me. Susi,
Matt and the girls are leaving Friday morning for

Tennessee to visit Matt's folks. Since they'll be away for a few days, we decided to buy the meat Susi can't bear to look at: lamb and calves liver. Remember? Since she moved here, Susi can't even think of eating her neighbors. Ronni is coming out to spend the weekend with us, and we're hoping the chemo won't have any uncomfortable results in the next few days. So far so good!

THURSDAY, AUGUST 2, 2007

Started the day with all the necessities: potassium through the tube, Ensure down the tube and a shot of Neupogen. And my patient is doing very well today. There are all kinds of secret meetings going on re: my surprise party. I've been very good and try to keep out of the way. The Wynn family plans to leave at 4 A.M. tomorrow for their Tennessee trip, so we'll wish them bon voyage tonight. I have been stalling on having a party. After Gerry's diagnosis, I wasn't sure he'd be here for it, but my boy is so strong mentally and so courageous, he'll come through with flying colors.

Friday, August 3, 2007

The Wynns left at 4 A.M. Grumpy started running at
4:15 A.M. Immodium fixed him up. Since his stomach
was iffy, I suggested that maybe we shouldn't have the
lamb shanks tonight. He said, in no uncertain terms,
"If I'm going to be sick, I may as well enjoy my dinner.
We're having lamb!" Ronni and Scott came out this
morning and they'll stay until Sunday. This afternoon
we went to a rental place to order a tent, tables and
chairs for my "surprise" party.

Saturday, August 4, 2007

Eric drove out today to see his Grumpy (and Grammy).
And guess what? We all went to a movie. The first
one for Gerry in four months. Saw "The Bourne
Ultimatum" and loved the action. Tonight the boys
are grilling chicken on our wonderful grill, and we're
having fresh corn from the local farm. So far, the
patient has been eating! Cousin Harriet called from
Florida to ask if I was practicing how to look surprised.
Don't think so, unless the gang comes up with
something I don't know about. Eric, Scott and I played
Boggle while Ronni kept her daddy company. He's a
little pooped after the movie trip.

SUNDAY, AUGUST 5, 2007

When I said Gerry was a little pooped, I didn't realize
how accurate that word was. He awoke at 2 A.M. with
the runs. By 8 A.M., he was O.K. and has been fine all
day. So, he wants liver and onions for dinner. Don't
know how smart that is, but we'll find out! Ronni
and boys left this afternoon and the house is so
quiet! Andrea called from Tennessee and said they
saw "Hairspray" today and loved it. Amy called from
Colorado to say she saw "Hairspray" today and loved
it. As soon as Grumpy feels up to it, maybe we can see
"Hairspray" and love it!!!

MONDAY, AUGUST 6, 2007

O.K. So liver and onions was not such a good idea.
It was delicious, but he started running like the
Energizer bunny at 2:30 A.M. and stopped at 8 A.M.
So far, so good! Maybe he'll behave when it comes to
the menu selection tonight. Had to have a new line
installed for our bedroom air conditioner. They said
they'd be here between 8 and 9 in the morning. After
being up a lot during the night, it was a challenge
getting out of bed at 7 A.M. But we did it! Flushed the
feeding tube, took our morning meds, got dressed, and
waited...and waited. Finally, at 9:30 the electrician
showed up. He did a good job, but we hate getting up
early when we don't have to. Got up early enough when
we were working folks!

Tuesday, August 7, 2007

Quiet today. Went to oncologist and Gerry's red count was a little low, so they gave him a procrit shot. Luckily, no transfusion necessary. His stomach is back to normal, so I wonder what he's planning for dinner. Dare I try liver and onions again? Ordered more Neupogen for next week's round of chemo. That means I get to shoot the patient 5 days in a row. I feel like Annie Oakley!

Wednesday, August 8, 2007

Went to pulmonary doctor today, and Gerry's chest infection has cleared up. He can stop antibiotics that he's been on for five weeks. The patient felt well enough to drive his nurse to the doctor and to the super market afterwards. What a luxury! The Wynns are due home tomorrow. Can't wait to see our gang. House is too quiet! There was a storm last night and we slept right through it. Turned on the TV this morning and saw pictures of devastation in New York and New Jersey, with no subways running and possible tornadoes in Brooklyn. Didn't hear a thing!

Thursday, August 9, 2007

The Wynn family was due to arrive midday today. At 6:30 A.M. we heard a voice saying, "We're home!" Seems they couldn't find a motel with vacancies, so Matt pulled over, slept for an hour and drove straight through. Gerry went for his PT evaluation this morning. They tested him to see what needs strengthening. Everything could use a little help. He has pages of exercises to do at home and will go to PT three times a week.

Friday, August 10, 2007

Crummy, rainy day today. Good time to go shopping. A few days ago when we were in Sam's Club, Gerry was pushing the cart with one hand and holding up his pants with the other hand. When we returned home, he walked into the bedroom and his pants fell down. He rushed to the scale and found that he has now lost 36 pounds! A helluva way to diet. So we went to look for shorts with elastic and draw string waists. Don't want them falling down in Sam's Club! Found shorts and a belt with grommet holes the whole length of the belt. This way, if he loses or gains weight, the clothes will always fit.

Saturday, August 11, 2007

Beautiful day today. Grumpy wore a pair of his new shorts with drawstring and they stayed up! Niece Sherry and nephew Jim visited today, and we enjoyed our usual killer game of dominoes. Gerry has had a good two days. Hopefully, we'll get to a movie tomorrow. Want to get it all in before chemo starts on Tuesday. Ronni is spending the weekend here while her men are on a canoe/camping trip on the Delaware River with their cousins and Mark's brother Freddie. Since she loves tuna casserole and nobody at her home will eat it, that's what I'm making for dinner!

Sunday, August 12, 2007

We decided to go to a morning movie today (cheaper!). Grumpy got up unwillingly, took his pills and almost went on strike. "My foot hurts and I'm staying home." I told him it would hurt whether he stayed home or went to the movies, so he might as well get out of the house and enjoy himself with his harem (Susi, Ronni, Nicole, Andrea and me). The pressure worked. He went with us to see "Hairspray" and we had a wonderful time, although Gerry and Ronni weren't quite as enthusiastic as we were about the film. Ronni left to get ready for her camper/canoers. Can't wait to hear about their adventure. Amy called to say they saw "Rush Hour 3" and loved it. Come to think of it, Amy loves most movies! Maybe that's the next one we'll drag Gerry to.

Monday, August 13, 2007

The Grumpster started PT today. They worked him over for an hour and a half and he did great! I thought he would be achy from the exercises, but I haven't heard one complaint. Tomorrow is chemo/date day. Amy called to say she was in the emergency room. Trouble breathing and that ain't good! Her asthma acted up during a 100-degree heat wave in Denver. During the heat wave, their swamp cooler broke (Colorado equivalent to air conditioning). Hard to breathe when there's no cool air anywhere in the house. She was dehydrated, and feels much better after getting intravenous liquids. And Amy is always walking around with water bottles. Go figure!

Tuesday, August 14, 2007

Gerry had his chemo visit today and all went well. Had his procrit shot in the office, and starting tomorrow I give him the Neupogen shots 5 days in a row. He was a little sore today from the PT yesterday, but I figure that's a good sign. The muscles are waking up. More PT tomorrow.

Wednesday, August 15, 2007

PT went very well today. Gerry learned how to get out of a chair without help, and that helps the nurse. No chemo next week because the doctor wants him to feel well for my surprise party on August 26. He'll start chemo after the party, and will probably have a cat scan in September.

Thursday, August 16, 2007

Shot Grumpy two days in a row. Good job, too. And here's some good news. Grumpy weighed himself this morning and he has gained nine pounds. He's eating a few meals a day instead of one big meal at night. This way, he's getting a lot more nourishment. Combined with the exercise regimen from PT, he's doing pretty damn good! We drove to Middletown today so Nicole could do her college dorm shopping. Good thing we have a mini van! Andrea got some stuff for high school while we were out, and we have two happy girls!

Friday, August 17, 2007

Bad weather today, so everyone is aching a little more than usual. But that didn't stop Gerry and Susi from going into town to do some shopping. Some of the shopping trip may have to do with my surprise next week, but as they say, "don't ask, don't tell."

Saturday, August 18, 2007

Susi and the girls left with Matt early this morning. He's going to work and they're going to see Les Miserable. Ronni came out this morning, and Gerry, Ronni and yours truly went to the movies. Yes! We saw Rush Hour 3 and it was a very funny film. After the movie date, we went to Friday's for lunch. First time we've been to a restaurant in months. Quite a remarkable day. Reminds you of every-day things you usually take for granted.

SUNDAY, AUGUST 19, 2007

After a full day yesterday, we're all pooped out today. Got an e-mail from cousin Bess in Virginia asking how many chemo treatments are left. We have no idea, but think it will be a long haul. As long as it shrinks the no-good cells, we're all for doing whatever it takes. Company coming from Florida tomorrow, our very dear friends Susan and Jerry. Susan went to school with our Susan, so we go back a long time!

MONDAY, AUGUST 20, 2007

Spending valuable time with Susan and Jerry. Having such a good time reminiscing and catching up.Gerry felt washed out yesterday, but is revived today. Company will do that for you. Andrea is walking around the house all day singing songs from Les Miz. Nicole keeps reminding Susi how many days are left before she leaves for college. Susi is trying not to think about it!

TUESDAY, AUGUST 21, 2007

Drove to Dr. K today and got a good report. In fact, she told Gerry he was getting boring. No challenges for her because things are going so well. She also told him he could drink beer at my surprise party this coming Sunday. He asked her if he could only drink it on Sunday, and she said it was O.K. to have one whenever he felt like it. Way to go, Doc! His red blood count was a little low, so she gave him a procrit shot. Gerry resumes chemo the Tuesday after the party. Then I get to shoot him five days in a row for the white count. Four more days until the Colorado gang arrives!

Phone rang early this morning. It was oncologist's office telling us that Gerry's potassium is low, so he gets the orange-colored liquid down the tube twice a day for three days. I called a piano tuner to tune the piano I've had since I was 8 years old. He was due around 10:15. Got a call from the party rental place, and they said they were delivering the tent today, a day early, since most of their employees were heading back to college. Piano tuner arrived first, and we told him to park on the lawn, since the driveway is where the tent is being set up for my big surprise bash. The tuning man got out of his car very slowly. He was VERY old. We helped carry his equipment, hoping he would make it up the steps to the living room. After a few hours, piano was tuned (per request from son-in-law Carl, our Colorado musician). We helped the Piano Man (no relation to Billy Joel) back to his car and I told him we were having a party for my 75th birthday. He said, "How old do you think I am?" I said, "80?" No, he said proudly. "I'm 93!" While he was tuning, the rental people arrived. What a big mother of a tent. 20 feet by 40 feet. Took them two hours to set up and to unload the tables and chairs. Looks like someone is having a party! While all this was taking place, Grumpy drove himself to PT. He promises to rest for a few days, so he'll be in good shape on Sunday.

THURSDAY, AUGUST 23, 2007

Interesting things going on around here. Gave Gerry his potassium down the tube, and then Gerry, Susi and I drove to Middletown. First stop was a party store. I was instructed to stay in the car while they went in to get some "stuff" for you-know-what. Next stop was Sam's Club, where we picked up a lot of nosh for the Wynn, Michelson and Hansen families...as well as for people coming by on Sunday for the big surprise. Cousin Harriet called to say she couldn't wait to see us on Saturday. Told her if she and Abe showed up on Saturday, it would be a day before the caterer arrived. Oops! When we came home from shopping trip, I was instructed to stay downstairs. Something is brewing upstairs and I will undoubtedly be surprised with whatever they're planning. The only thing I have planned is a song in the key of G (whoever is playing the guitar, please note). Two more days till Colorado clan arrives. Getting very excited, especially every time I look out of the window and see the enormous tent in the driveway!

Friday, August 24, 2007

Two days till the big day, and things are really hopping! Got a beautiful bouquet of flowers delivered today from dear friends, Nick and Annie, who lived across the street from us in Florida. Even if it was a surprise, the flowers and tent in the driveway would have given it away! Gerry Boy was his usual smart-aleck self this morning. I was sitting at the computer and he walked in and said, "Either your hair is crooked or your head is." The dear was referring to my braid, which is sometimes off-center. Is that any way to treat Nurse Ratched?

Saturday, August 25, 2007

Things are getting exciting! Today a beautiful bouquet arrived from Joel and Diane in Mill Valley, CA. Ronni and Scott came out early and the gang set up tables under the tent. So impressive! Eric is driving out tomorrow, and Mark is picking up the Colorado gang at Newark Airport. Amy just called to say the eagle has landed. She was a little nervous after watching news stories about near misses at airports. Gerry is resting today, getting ready for the mob scene tomorrow. He weighed himself today, and he gained two more pounds. Yeah! Got a real surprise tonight when the whole gang gathered to give me pre-birthday presents. The kids and grandkids gave me a collection of folk-song DVD's and a book on the history of folk singing. Gerry gave me a beautiful diamond circle necklace. The jeweler said it was called the circle of life, but Gerry said it was the circle of love. What a special guy!

Sunday, August 26, 2007

Someone just walked by with dozens of balloons, but I didn't see them (ha ha). Catering truck just arrived, but I'm not allowed outside until they give me permission. Aren't surprise parties fun? The Grumpster is resting now before the party begins, so he can mingle later. I decided to put on makeup for the occasion. Since I haven't worn it in ages, and since it's a mad house here today, I hurried through the process and thought I did a good job. Then Amy walked in and said I looked like a Vulcan (Spock eyebrows from Star Trek). Amy and Ronni both brushed and smudged and whatever you're supposed to do, so now I look like an old broad who is part of the Earth people. Gerry took a fall right before the party began, and cut his arm and bruised other limbs. The kids picked him up and I wiped the blood off Grumpy while Nicole wiped Grumpy's blood off Scott's shirt. Bad dress rehearsal is good performance, right? Will talk all about it tomorrow. Just too tired to write tonight.

Well, the surprise came and went and it was wonderful! Even the weather was wonderful, after they forecast thunderstorms and the sun came out. About 80 relatives and friends joined in this incredible day. Ronni sang a beautiful song that she composed for her parents. She wrote both music and lyrics and we have it on a CD to preserve that special moment. Nicole got up and apologized for singing, and then sang a song she wrote to a Simon and Garfunkel tune. A little off-key, but no need for apology. It was terrific! Then I sang a song I wrote for my own bash...thanking Gerry Boy for my surprise party The caterer did a superb job. Barbecued everything on the spot and had side dishes galore. Susi and the girls made center pieces for all the tables, as well as a picture board containing pix of Little Audrey up to older Audrey, as well as a memory book containing pictures, poems and sayings from so many people! Gerry held a special place of honor. He couldn't really table hop, so he sat on a comfortable chair while everyone visited with him. And he lasted the whole day...until late in the evening. That was the icing on the cake. Talking of icing on the cake, the cake had my picture on it, taken from the invitation. Problem with that is, when they cut into the cake, they cut off my head. I felt like Marie Antoinette!

TUESDAY, AUGUST 28, 2007

Today was chemo/date day. We packed our lunch
and our books and drove to Middletown. They took
a blood sample, came in and said, "No chemo today.
Your platelet count is too low." A very disappointed
Gerry drove back home...happy to see his family, but
unhappy about not getting the treatment. Evidently,
there's nothing you can do to raise the platelet count
(which the chemo reduces). They don't give platelet
transfusions unless it is very low, so we'll wait till next
week and hope it rises. You think yeast would help?
Mark and Eric left yesterday, Ronni and Scott left
today, and we spent the afternoon watching "Blades
of Glory." Had more fun watching Ryan's face than
watching the movie. There were some parts that were
not too appropriate, and he loved every minute of it!!!

WEDNESDAY, AUGUST 29, 2007

Well, it's official. I'm 75 today! Amy told me I didn't
look a day over 74. In fact, when Amy arrived, she
walked into Gerry's room and said, "Gee, you don't look
as bad as I thought you would!" Cute kid! Gerry brought
his mini van in for service yesterday because he wasn't
happy with the air conditioning. He had a right not to
be happy. We picked it up today, and they had to replace
the compressor (we thought it was only the coolant).

Good thing this expense occurred after my party! The patient's arms and hands look like Jackson Pollack paintings...all splattered in red. Every time he knocks into something, these strange things appear on his skin. That's because the platelet count is so low. Sure hope it's high enough for chemo next week.

Thursday, August 30, 2007

Today I am one year younger than Gerry. Tomorrow I'll be two years younger. Isn't that amazing? The Grumpster celebrates number 77 tomorrow. Here's to 120! Carl visited his mom in Vermont for two days and came back today, just in time to cook three dinners for us. He leaves this Sunday, but promises a feast every night. Gerry had PT today, and did very well. He lifted two-pound weights with his hands, and that's a lot when you've lost so much muscle tone. The kids are having a grand time with their Colorado kin. A lot happening in next few days. Eric and Scott leave for college Saturday, Nicole leaves on Monday. Andrea enters high school Tuesday. Ryan had already started 4th Grade before the trip East, but he reads every day to catch up with his school mates.

Friday, August 31, 2007

Gerry is a birthday boy today. Carl made a special
brunch for the occasion. Pancakes from scratch,
scrambled eggs with cheese and sausage. He ate it
all without any swallowing trouble! Yeah! We had a
birthday celebration, and our Gerry Boy got cards
and gifts and lots of hugs!

Saturday, September 1, 2007

Beautiful day today. Amy's friend Sue, from high
school days, came to visit. Amazing how they still look
like teenagers! Gerry, Carl and I went shopping to get
food for tonight and tomorrow. Tonight Carl is making
beer butt chicken on the grill. I think polite people
call it beer can chicken. Carl leaves tomorrow and
Grumpy is planning to drive him to the airport. Way
to go, Gerry! Tomorrow Gerry is also planning to grill
steak for Nicole's good-bye dinner, and that girl LOVES
steak! I'll be making the wine and mushroom sauce to
go with it. Back to tonight's dinner. Gerry was looking
forward to it all week. Beer butt chicken, Caesar salad,
spare ribs, fresh corn from the farm, grilled zucchini.
He sat down, took a bite of spareribs and a taste of
salad and all of a sudden he was in terrible pain. Food
didn't go down. Since he missed chemo last week, we
fear that something may have returned. After about
three hours, he felt fine again, but we're all concerned.

SUNDAY, SEPTEMBER 2, 2007

Today Gerry is eating again...very carefully. Today
Ronni came out, and Gerry, Ronni, Amy and I drove
Carl to Newark Airport. First time the patient has
driven for over an hour in four months, and he was a
real champ! Right now Matt and Ryan are mowing the
lawn. Ryan is so excited about steering a power mower.
Gerry and gang are on the deck cleaning the grill,
getting ready for Nicole's steak dinner tonight. Susi
and Nicole are packing everything the college
girl will need, since tomorrow is the big day! Andrea
is doing her best to keep Gerry's spirits up. She
does a platelet dance every day. "Wazzup? Platelets!"
Hopefully, he'll get chemo on Tuesday. Ryan was a little
antsy at bedtime. Amy told him he had to settle down
and he said, "Mom, I have restless body syndrome."

MONDAY, SEPTEMBER 3, 2007

Gerry is still having trouble swallowing. Not to
worry. Nurse Ratched is here to take care of him. This
morning I was pouring Ensure down the tube after
his shower. While I was pouring, Gerry was watching
a cooking show on the Food Channel. All of a sudden
he said, "Look at this!" So I looked, and I poured the
Ensure all over his chest. Oops! In the meantime,
it's soup, pudding, apple sauce and down-the-tube
Ensure. Niece Sherry and nephew Jim called to say that
the DVD they took at my surprise party came out well.
They're trying to figure out how to make copies.

Good project for Labor Day. Nicole went to college today. Boo hoo. Miss her already. Carl made it back to Colorado safely, and since Eric and Scott are both back at Rutgers, Ronni left this morning to join Mark in the empty nest.

Good news! Platelet count doubled since last week. Chemo date is on. Andrea gave Grumpy her old iPod, which he brought with him today. I was busy reading and he was busy keeping time with his hands and feet (while in the chair with chemo dripping). All of a sudden a booming voice started singing Besame Mucho...in the key of Off. Because of the earphones, he didn't realize how loud he was. Everyone got a big kick out of him. We were hoping to get chemo date for next week, but doctor sticks to a strict schedule. Every third week is doctor's visit. After next week's visit with Doctor K, we'll be back to the two straight weeks of chemo.

Grumpy had PT this morning and is doing quite well. He still can't swallow real food, only liquids. So while he was doing his exercises, I went to the market and bought all the ingredients for chicken noodle matzo ball soup. My matzo balls are so fluffy, even problem swallowers can eat them! Andrea loves high school, and Nicole, Eric and Scott are loving college. I started shooting the patient today (Neupogen). We almost forgot, and only remembered when Gerry said his windshield wipers needed cleaning. I told him to use the alcohol squares I use for his shots. Oooh. Shots! So he got shot a few hours late!

Thursday, September 6, 2007

Gerry drove Amy, Ryan and me to Middletown today. The Colorado kid was getting bored with his cousins all in school. He got some neat clothes for his return to Fourth Grade. Grumpy got a new pair of jeans. I remembered to shoot the patient this morning. He still hasn't tried any solid foods, so it's boiled eggs, Ensure, pudding and ice cream diet. His mood is very positive, even if Andrea calls him an old poop (have to show her the movie "On Golden Pond"...where that expression comes from).

Friday, September 7, 2007

Grumpy bought himself a new radio alarm clock. Pretty snazzy. You can even point a projector to the ceiling to see the time during the night. Trouble is, we thought we knew how to set it, but it didn't go off this morning. Almost missed PT. Gerry had his evaluation and is O.K. to get therapy for another four weeks. This afternoon we plan to read the alarm clock instruction book. Doh! The jeans that Gerry bought yesterday fit so well, we drove back to Middletown today to get two more pair. Since the weight loss, the boy needs pants that won't fall down. Nicole came home for the weekend and helped with the shopping.

SATURDAY, SEPTEMBER 8, 2007

Today is the last day of Amy's and Ryan's visit. Have
to get a lot of hugs today! Gerry is still on his liquid-
ish diet, but can down pudding, ice cream and an
occasional black and white cookie. The Michelson clan
is celebrating Rutgers win over Navy last night.
Go Scarlet Knights!

SUNDAY, SEPTEMBER 9, 2007

Quite a day. Susi and Matt took Nicole back to college.
Gerry was supposed to drive Amy and Ryan to the
airport, but this morning he started running like the
Energizer bunny. Forgot to mention that last night he
ate real food for the first time in days: shrimp cocktail,
pasta and biscuits. Maybe that's what did him in. I
drove Amy and Ryan to the airport, and Andrea joined
me for the ride. My sidekick on the way home. Gerry
said Amy called from the airport to say there was a
lockdown in one area and thousands of people were
crowding around, not knowing what to do or where to
go. Even the Captain and crew had trouble getting to
the gate, but she called back a little while later to say
they were on the plane!

Monday, September 10, 2007

Amy and Ryan arrived home safely last night. I
followed them on the internet site until they landed.
Gerry was a little washed out from yesterday's episode,
so he cancelled PT today. Tomorrow we visit Doctor K
and we'll see what's next. He's swallowing a little better
and will try to eat some dinner tonight. The patient is
rebelling against the soft-food diet.

Tuesday, September 11, 2007

Grumpy woke up today feeling much better. Went to
oncologist and got a good report. He has chemo again
next Tuesday and follow-up chemo the Tuesday after.
Then comes the cat scan to tell us how it's going. After
the scan, she may stay with the same regimen or
change it. The boy is starting to eat real food again,
and that helps the spirit. When we were talking about
my surprise party with the doctor, and she said that
Gerry could have a beer, he mentioned that he liked
Heineken Light. She said she never tasted it. So today
we brought her two bottles of the brew and she gave out
a big grin! Guess she'll drink it after hours. Strange
day today, remembering 9-11. Our thoughts are with
everyone who lost a loved one, and a nation that lost its
innocence. Here's to better days ahead.

WEDNESDAY, SEPTEMBER 12, 2007

Another day in Pine Island…land of the black dirt
farms. Got a call from oncologist today, telling us
that Grumpy's potassium was a little low. So I pour
potassium down the tube twice a day for two days.
He felt well enough to go to PT, but when he finished
the exercises, he made a mad dash to the bathroom.
Energizer bunny kicked in again and he started
running. That happens sometimes with the potassium.
We're hoping it's a one-shot deal and he can resume
eating again. The boy does love to eat real food. I'll
be cooking tomorrow for the holidays, and he'll be
eating away no matter how he feels. Chicken soup
can only help!

THURSDAY, SEPTEMBER 13, 2007

Happy New Year to everyone celebrating today
(Rosh Hashanah). We celebrated by visiting the
rheumatologist. I got a shot in the knee and Gerry
got a shot in the shoulder. We seem to do everything
together. Talking about doing things together, I also
got an RX for PT. Maybe that will help this old knee
from hurting. Amy told me about a series of three shots
called Synvisc. It's made from chickens, or turkeys,
or Cornish hens…some poultry. If PT doesn't work,
doctor will give me the Synvisc option. House smells
wonderful with the aroma coming from the crock pot:
pot roast for tomorrow's company. Matzo ball soup

will be made tomorrow, and if Gerry can't eat the pot roast, there'll be loads of matzo balls and noodles for him. Today the boy is doing pretty well, considering a couple of lousy days. He's looking forward to chemo on Tuesday, our date day.

Friday, September 14, 2007

All the family is here except the Colorado contingent, who are here in spirit. Gerry couldn't eat the pot roast, but was delighted to have a big portion of matzo ball soup and a small portion of peach noodle pudding. Beats Ensure down the tube!

Saturday, September 15, 2007

The Michelsons left early this afternoon. They wanted to get home in time to watch the Rutgers football game on TV. It's now half time and Rutgers is winning 45-0. Yeah team! The girls in this house couldn't care less about football or any other sport. They are all into Broadway musicals and latest CD's and DVD's. Personally, I'd rather hear Andrea sing than hear an announcer shouting football stats. It was such a strange day today, we forgot it was Saturday and forgot to pick up the mail at out post office. Guess the bills will have to wait until Monday. Back to the second half!

SUNDAY, SEPTEMBER 16, 2007

Quiet day today. Matt is mowing the lawn and Grumpy is watching football games. He warns me that there is more football tonight, so I'll be watching HGTV in the next room. Susi and Matt are bringing Nicole back to school in a little while. Andrea will hang out with the Old Poops (as she lovingly calls us). Tomorrow Gerry has PT and Tuesday he has chemo. The boy is in good spirits and looking forward to eating some real foods again. In fact, he tried some herring in sour cream sauce and enjoyed every bit!

MONDAY, SEPTEMBER 17, 2007

A real autumn day here today. We brought our mini van in for some body work. Want the outside to stay as good as the inside. From there we went to PT to take care of Grumpy's body works. He's doing pretty well, considering he hasn't eaten real food in a few days. He can't wait to start chemo tomorrow so he can eat again! My knee felt great for one and a half days after being shot. Now it's back to Lidocaine patches and limping. Some nurse!

Tuesday, September 18, 2007

Had our chemo date today. All the counts were up.
Guess the platelet dance helped. Wazzup? Platelets!
Seven hours of relaxation. Read books, ate lunch and
kibbutzed with the nurses. Tomorrow Nurse Ratched
gets to shoot the patient again...five days straight.
All Gerry wants now is to eat real food. Hoping he can
start to swallow in a day or two.

Wednesday, September 19, 2007

Fun day today. Started off by shooting Gerry with
Neupogen. Then we stopped at Orange Regional
Medical Center to pick up two bottles of "stuff" that he
has to drink next Wednesday before the cat scan. Then
onto Macy's — where the boy got two sweat suit outfits
for the cold weather a-coming. Then we picked up the
mini van that was just repaired. Looks like new! Since
chemo yesterday, patient has been able to swallow a
little better. Yippee! Miracle poison!

Thursday, September 20, 2007

Gerry went to PT today and did 22-1/2 minutes on the
treadmill. Then we went to Macy's to get more "stuff."
The sweat suits we got yesterday were too small. Gerry
thought size Large would be more than adequate, with
all the weight he lost, but he needed that XL size. Then
we stopped at Lazy Boy to see if they could add a lift
to the swivel rocker we bought last year. The seat and
arms of the chair are way too low, and the patient has
difficulty getting out of it. Since the chair swivels

and rocks, we were told it was dangerous to add a platform. We then checked out an electric chair...not the kind they use for murderers...the one that lifts you up and out. Since the price tag is very steep, we think we'll shop around.

Friday, September 21, 2007

The Grumpster had his third shot this morning. Two more to go for Nurse Ratched until next week, when I get to shoot him again. He ate a little chopped liver for lunch and had no problems. Good omen. I spent the afternoon preparing goodies for tomorrow night's meal. Gerry spent the afternoon in front of the TV watching cooking shows. He's preparing himself for the time when he can eat again. Guess I should mention that while I was preparing devilled eggs, my right thumb went into a trigger-like position and I couldn't move it. Hurts like hell, besides being crooked. So I stuffed the eggs with my left hand and left them for Susi to put away. She came downstairs and asked me why the eggs looked so cockeyed. I promised to let her know next time one of my fingers cramps up. So we're having cockeyed devilled eggs tomorrow.

Saturday, September 22, 2007

Today is Yom Kippur, the Day of Atonement. The Michelsons joined us today, and they all fasted. It was worth the wait for the goodies that followed at sundown. Grumpy, who has almost been fasting for the last few weeks, ate a real supper: lox, soft onion roll, homemade potato salad, cockeyed devilled eggs, noodle pudding, herring in cream sauce, white fish, sable, etc. What a pleasure to see him eat! Sherry and Jim spent the day here, and we followed the meal with our usual bang-up game of Dominoes.

Sunday, September 23, 2007

Today was an eventful day. We bought an electric chair. Once Gerry sits down, he pushes a button to recline and pushes another to lift him into an almost-standing position. Amy and Carl suggested that we put a metal colander on his head with wires sticking out, so it looks like the real electric chair, but we declined the sicko idea (though I do love dark humor). It will be delivered Thursday, and the patient can't wait! All our college kiddoes returned to school today. Andrea has two friends from drama club visiting, and Gerry and I are enjoying the sounds of music emanating from upstairs.

Monday, September 24, 2007

Today we had a PT date. Ain't love grand? I actually felt
better when we left, and the Gerry Boy did 22 minutes
on the treadmill. We are making calls to find someone
to remove our love seat before the electric chair
arrives. Tuesday is chemo. Wednesday is cat scan.
Busy week coming up!

Tuesday, September 25, 2007

Had our chemo date today. Platelets were a little
low, but not low enough to stop the procedure. Yeah!
Nicole charged the iPod so Grumpy could zone out
and sing off key. Problem is, we forgot to bring it. I
put it in our "chemo bag" when we got home so it won't
happen again. Tomorrow is cat scan day. Have to go to
a different hospital earlier to get his blood checked...
to make sure everything is up to par for the "pictures."
Guess we'll do a cat scan dance tonight!

Wednesday, September 26, 2007

Guess the cat scan dance worked. Because some
levels in his blood were a little high, they did the
scan without contrast. Not quite as thorough as with
contrast, but hopefully, it will be good enough to see
the good results. Gerry only wanted to stop at Nathan's
on the way home for a hot dog and fries, but figured
he'd wait until next week, when he plans to be eating
again. Tomorrow is electric chair day. They called to
say they would be here between 7 and 11 A.M. Oy!

That means we have to roll out of bed mighty early so I can pour water down the tube, shoot the patient with Neupogen, get dressed and be ready for the big event. I re-arranged what I could in the living room, because the chair has to be near an electric source. Don't want anyone (like moi) to trip while walking by.

Thursday, September 27, 2007

Today is the big electric chair day. It was due to arrive between 7 and 11 A.M., so we were up at 6:30 (yawn). Chair was delivered at 10:30 and we loved it. Tried the reclining and standing positions while the delivery men were here and it worked perfectly. Susi was not home when the chair arrived, so when she returned, I told Grumpy to demonstrate his new toy. He sat down, pushed the DOWN bottom and reclined. Then he pushed the UP button, and nothing happened. Friggin' chair was frozen in the down position. Susi and I both had to help Gerry out of the chair. Called the store and they said they'd send somebody tomorrow. I told them "not good enough." So the delivery men came back at 7 P.M. Tried all the tricks and chair wouldn't budge. They took it away and we'll call the store tomorrow to arrange for a new one. Do you think it was made in China?

Friday, September 28, 2007

Seems we do everything together. This morning was
a visit to the podiatrist. This afternoon we went to
PT. Grumpy had quite a workout on the treadmill and
other machines. He's such a brave guy! I just did knee
exercises. Ouch! Now for the friggin' chair saga. A new
one will be delivered next Wednesday. Nicole is coming
home for the weekend and expects to see Gerry's new
toy, but she'll have to wait until next weekend.

Saturday, September 29, 2007

Not a good day for Grumpy. Having some trouble
swallowing pills and food. He was able to eat a fish dish
tonight: tilapia rolled up and baked in a mushroom/
wine sauce. He was more upset with the Rutgers game
than the food problem. We both screamed at the TV,
but they lost anyway!

Sunday, September 30, 2007

Gerry is doing a little better today. Had a croissant
with cheese spread for breakfast and grilled cheese
and tomato sandwich for lunch. Problem is, the nurse
tried Pam instead of butter and burned one side of
the cheese sandwich. He ate in anyway. That's how
desperate he is for food! Matt was busy, so Gerry, Susi,
Andrea and I drove Nicole back to SUNY Purchase.
First time we've seen her dorm. Nice room! Her
roommate who never speaks was not there, not that
it would have mattered. Grumpy had quite a workout
getting to the dorm. A very healthy walk that included

steps. By time we got to Nicole's room, he felt like he had two hours of therapy. There was a parking lot right next to the dorm for students and teachers with passes, and we didn't realize we could have parked there. So Susi and I shlepped back to the car and picked the patient up. Just got back home and guess what? He's watching football!

MONDAY, OCTOBER 1, 2007

Well, today was a strange one. Grumpy wasn't feeling well — stomach hurt, chest hurt, back of neck hurt. Called the oncologist and asked if we could come in today instead of tomorrow. Good thing. First of all, she said the results of the cat scan showed that he was stable, but she believes that an inflammation of the pancreas is causing the discomfort. She also said he was going directly from her office to the hospital, where he will remain with IV's etc. until the pancreas has a chance to calm down. He's in Arden Hill Hospital, and will be there a few days or longer, depending upon how he reacts to the treatments. I had to run home to bring back pajamas and all that stuff and got lost both ways. Nothing like taking the scenic route!

Great news! Susi and I went to the hospital this morning and Gerry was in a very good mood (think it was the pain meds?).The nurse came in to say the doctor wants him to try to eat some lunch. The food came, and it was probably the worst food anyone has ever consumed. The nurses were ordering Chinese food for lunch, so he put in his order for egg drop soup. He ate a little and made an amazing discovery. His neck, that was giving him so much pain these last few weeks, felt fine! Susi gave him a foot massage and the Grumpster said, "Who could ask for anything better? ME!" Little did he know that better things were in store. The scopes and scans came out perfect. They think he had this pancreatitis for a few weeks, and it was now calming down. Blood tests showed no signs of danger, so we kissed the patient good night and headed home. A nurse gave me directions and this time I did it! I told Susi to call Gerry to tell him we were almost by the house and were going to the gas station. Gerry told Susi the doctor was just in and had just left. He also said the doctor said he could go home tonight. So we picked up Andrea, turned the car around and headed back to ye olde hospital. Took about an hour and a half to get him released, but Grumpy is home and happy, and we're happy to have our darling with us. Tomorrow, the electric chair comes again.

WEDNESDAY, OCTOBER 3, 2007

The electric chair has arrived! They said between 7
A.M. and noon. By 12: 30 I was getting nervous, but
at 12:45 the friggin' chair arrived. It's been seven
minutes now, and it still works! Considering the last
two days, the patient is in good shape. A little tired
from the hospital experience, but in very good spirits.
Susi was out shopping when chair arrived and she
just walked in. Gerry demonstrated his new toy with
trepidation, and hallelujah – it works!!!

THURSDAY, OCTOBER 4, 2007

Electric chair is still working. It was so comfortable,
Grumpy spent most of the day sleeping in it. Today
he said, "Enough is enough!" So first he helped Susi
rearrange the large pantry closet in the kitchen. We
can now actually find the food! And then he drove me
to Sam's Club to pick up a few goodies. Nicole comes
home tonight for the week-end. Tomorrow is Andrea's
15th birthday. Hard to believe! I remember when she
was 14. Susi is taking her to see "Spring Awakening"
on Broadway Saturday. Matt is taking Nicole to see the
86th Street Subway Station in Manhattan for an art
project. Giving Gerry Ensure Plus now, so he'll have
extra protein. Has to be vanilla, because Stanley told
him it tasted good (even though I'm pouring it down
the tube). Go figure!

Friday, October 5, 2007

Our Andrea is 15 today. She opened her gifts right after school. If she waited for Matt to come home from work, her birthday would practically be over (he gets home around 9 P.M. every night). Our friend/neighbor Eve visited today, and we had lots of funny stories to share. Eve is director of the Black Dirt Dance Studio where Gerry and I took yoga classes and Susi and I took belly dancing. Those were the days before feeding tubes and bum knees. Nice day today. Wild turkeys in the backyard, each the size of an emu. Strange creatures. Not your usual Thanksgiving fare. Nicole took pix of Gerry in his electric chair (complete with colander on his head to look more authentic). Susi is posting them tonight on the Caring Bridge web site.

Saturday, October 6, 2007

The Wynns left for their New York City trip this morning. Ronni came out and had a splendid idea. Since we bought a DVD burner a while back and only transferred three tapes, she started burning some of the old family treasures. Only have about 100 to go, Grumpy showed Ronni how to operate the machine and she was on a roll. I can't even figure out how to use the DVD player!

SUNDAY, OCTOBER 7, 2007

Grumpy is sitting in his electric chair "throne," yelling
at the TV while watching interceptions. Giving him
lots of Ensure between meals to keep his strength up.
Ronni made more DVD's from our tape collection. It's
such fun watching old movies of kids and grandkids
come to life. Andrea loved "Spring Awakening" and
Nicole got to take pictures of the 86th Street Subway
Station without getting in trouble with Homeland
Security. Apple Fest is going on in Warwick today.
That's a yearly event that draws about 30,000 people to
town, so Ronni will go home early tomorrow.

MONDAY, OCTOBER 8, 2007

What a lazy day! Ronni stayed until the afternoon to
help Nurse Ratched. She even did the feeding tube
without spilling Ensure all over the patient. This
afternoon we decided to watch a movie called "Babel."
Watched it for 2-1/2 hours and still don't know what
happened! I like final conclusions, not ones that
keep you hanging. Tomorrow we visit Dr. K to discuss
Gerry's next course of treatment.

Long day today. Went to oncologist for a visit. Gerry's blood count was a little low, so they gave him a procrit shot. Dr. K asked him if he'd like a transfusion before he begins chemo again next week. Since transfusions usually perk him up, he said YES! Went to the hospital to get his blood cross-checked the day before the vampires get him. He got a chest X-ray while we were there (shouldn't be a total loss). Doctor K is changing his chemo to a new recipe. He will be receiving Taxotere, instead of Cisplatin and CPT11. He'll get this once a week for three weeks, followed by doctor's appointment on fourth week. She said side effects should be mild. With this chemo, he doesn't need Neupogen any more, so I can't shoot the patient! (with all this shooting experience, I could have been governor of Alaska!). By time we got done with all the tests it was 4 P.M. and we were starving. So we went out to lunch. Haven't done that in ages, Went to Ruby Tuesday and ordered mini hamburgers. They weren't so mini, and we each got four of them! So we each ate one and brought six home. But it was so nice to go out to a restaurant!

WEDNESDAY, OCTOBER 10, 2007

Busy day. I had an early eye doctor appointment so we
would be on time for the transfusion at the hospital.
Arrived at the bloody place where the good vampires
hang out, and Gerry was hooked up for four hours.
When he was through, he was full of pep. In fact, he
was so strong, he wanted to go shopping at Macy's. So
off we went to buy a pair of suspenders. He's never
worn them (except with his tux), but has a problem
keeping his pants up. Because of the feeding tube,
he has to keep waist line lower than usual. So now he
looks like Larry King!

THURSDAY, OCTOBER 11, 2007

Went to pulmonologist today and brought Gerry's
X-rays taken on Tuesday. Lungs look pretty good except
for a little liquid at the bottom of the left one. Nothing
to be concerned about, says the doctor. Gerry has
been coughing a lot lately, and this is due to a sinus
infection. He is now on an antibiotic which should take
care of the matter. Tomorrow we are planning to go to
the Michelsons for the weekend. First two-hour trip in
six months. Better start packing all the gear needed for
Nurse Ratched to do her job properly. Gerry is wearing
his suspenders, and his pants stayed up all day!

Friday, October 12, 2007

Trip was great. Grumpy drove, but he had trouble getting up the few steps to Ronni's house. Ronni and I got on each side and acted as railings, and he finally got settled. Next problem: commode was way too low, so we went out and bought one with handles. Great for Gerry, but when I tried it, I felt like Lily Tomlin …only 3-1/2 years old. My feet didn't touch the floor (don't tell anyone, but when I tried it during the night, I peed all over the floor.) Now I move the contraption when it's my turn to use the bathroom. Mark made a delicious dinner, and Mark, Scott and Gerry spent the evening watching football on their new hi-def TV. With hi-def, you could see every blade of grass on the field!

Saturday, October 13, 2007

Had a good night and a good day. Watched Rutgers win on hi-def. Ronni and Mark went to a charity boat ride, formal clothes and all that jazz. They looked very snazzy. Friends Claire and Marty came over and we ordered in Japanese food, which Gerry was able to eat. Our two Rutgers grandsons, Eric and Scott, stayed home to join the "old folks."

Sunday, October 14, 2007

Today was football day. Again. Ronni and I stopped one game for two hours to watch a movie with Grumpy. Of course, it was a football movie: "We Are Marshall." Gerry is doing very well except for getting out of low chairs without handles. Mark taught us how to lift him up and now we are professionals. Mark took the college boys home tonight and we go home tomorrow.

Monday, October 15, 2007

Gerry planned on driving home, but when he got into the driver's seat, his foot was too swollen to lift onto the pedals. We call him Big Foot. Called the doctor when we returned home (about 2:30 P.M.) and she prescribed a diuretic. Tomorrow he starts the new chemo, if everything is a go. "Wazzup? Platelets!" Doing the chant today.

Tuesday, October 16, 2007

Started the new chemo today. Nicole's and Andrea's platelet chant worked. Count was way up! This is a much easier procedure. Only 2-1/2 hours instead of 6-7 hours. They say the after-effects are much milder, too. Let's hope! Big Foot still has a lot of fluid in his feet and legs. Couldn't lift them to drive today. Nurse Ratched is getting a lot of exercise lifting weights...the weights being those heavy feet that I lift onto the bed daily.

Andrea had a superb idea last night. Hang Gerry from the ceiling upside down so the water leaves the legs. What sympathy the patient is getting! We're preparing for a visit this weekend from my California brother and sister-in-law, the two most wonderful hippies you'd ever want to meet. Counting the days!

WEDNESDAY, OCTOBER 17, 2007

Very quiet day today. No doctors. No chemo. Susi and Grumpy are into the "Shield" series. I watched a few episodes with them today and can see how you get hooked. Amy and Sherry have a new chant: "Platelets up. Swelling down." Couldn't wait to see The Price Is Right with Drew Carey. Instead , there was a press conference with "W." He took away my favorite show!

THURSDAY, OCTOBER 18, 2007

Today Nurse Ratched had an eye doctor appointment. Since they had to dilate my eyes, Susi drove me to the visit. When she and Nicole picked me up two hours later, I was outside, wearing some strange looking glasses. Nicole said I looked like Ray Charles. So much for empathy. We wanted to go over some legal stuff with our attorney. I called to say that we had a slight problem. His office is up a big flight of stairs, and Big Foot can't handle the steps yet. He said that was no problem. He makes house calls. That's what happens when you live in the country. This wonderful man is coming at 5 P.M., and Grumpy can talk business while relaxing in his electric chair.

What a day! Susi, Nicole and I went grocery shopping for the company expected this weekend. Came back, opened the garage door, and saw water dripping from the light bulb over Susi's car. Susi ran upstairs and found the guest bathroom flooded. That's what was leaking down below. Couldn't figure out how to stop the flood, when Susi noticed the toilet tank was cracked. Guess after 25 years of service, it had enough. Susi called an emergency plumbing service. He told us to turn off the water from the house and he'd be here ASAP. A couple of hours later the plumber arrived, complete with a new toilet. One emergency averted. While all this was going on, I took Grumpy for a hair cut. He lost a lot of hair with the chemo (bye bye, braid) and what was left was standing up. He looked sort of like Einstein. Now he has a very neat trim, including what's left of his beard. Such a gorgeous guy! Denise, our favorite Pine Island hairdresser takes Gerry into her shop at a moment's notice. Everybody loves Gerry!

Ronni got here earlier and fed Gerry his lunch through the tube. She did very well! In the meantime, the bathroom leak saga continues. I went out to get the mail and noticed Susi's car covered with cardboard, and the ceiling opened up to dry. I thought Matt the Roofer did it. Mentioned it to Nicole, saying "I wonder why he didn't pull Susi's car out of the garage before he took down the ceiling." She looked at me, exasperated and said, "Grandma, Daddy didn't do that. The ceiling fell down!" I'm not a reliable witness. We took the soaked ceiling pieces off the car and Susi moved it into the driveway. The girls washed the car down and Susi told me she had a new theme song for the way this week has been going. From the show "Spring Awakening": Totally F***ed!! Mark, Eric and Scott are due to arrive shortly, and limo is picking up Joel and Diane around 5 P.M.

SUNDAY, OCTOBER 21, 2007

Great visit with Joel, Diane and the Michelson clan last night. They went to a nearby motel and we went to sleep. In the middle of the night, Grumpy woke up saying, "I'm soaked!" The J-tube entry into his stomach was leaking. Therefore, the bed was wet, his pajamas were soaked, etc. Changed the patient, the linens, and redid the tube, adding extra gauze pads to the opening. We slept fine the rest of the night. When Susi came down in the morning, we told her the story and she said, "Enough with the leaks in this house!" Pretty funny, considering yesterday's house damage. Great visit today. Had an early dinner, which Mark barbecued, and the Michelson men left at 5 P.M. Ronni is staying until Tuesday morning, and she is chauffeuring Joel and Diane to and from motel. Such a fun evening upstairs. With the help of the kids and grandkids, Gerry was able to make it up and down two days in a row! He even did a dance on the landing!

MONDAY, OCTOBER 22, 2007

Good night last night. Gerry was afraid that his
tube would leak again, but all was O.K. Will find out
tomorrow what happened when we visit the oncologist.
Second chemo of the new recipe, and so far so good.
Having such a wonderful time with Joel and Diane.
They'll be leaving tomorrow for the Big Apple and will
return to Mill Valley on Thursday.

TUESDAY, OCTOBER 23, 2007

Just got back from our chemo date. Doctor took a look
at Big Foot and said it wasn't an easy answer. When
either the heart, liver or kidneys are off, edema occurs.
In Gerry's case, it's the liver that still has some cancer
cells. Hopefully, the new chemo will shrink them.
She suggested that we get special socks with light
compression to help alleviate the swelling. Went to our
surgical supply store and bought three pairs of socks.
Two are easy to get on and one will probably break
my fingers, but hey, they don't call me Nurse Ratched
for nothing! Gerry put on the easier pair in the store.
Since he was wearing shorts and knee-highs, he looked
like a boy scout when he left. But the platelet dance
worked. Last month it was down to 75,000. Today the
count was 245,000. Yes!

WEDNESDAY, OCTOBER 24, 2007

Such a lazy day! Rain on and off and temperature is in the 50's. Have gotten used to summer weather, but can't complain. Called office of doctor who inserted the feeding tube and asked for an appointment for the Gerry Boy. The receptionist said the first available date in Goshen was November 12. I said, "That's not acceptable. His tube has been leaking and he needs an earlier appointment." She asked if we could go to his office in Monroe (an extra 10 minutes of drive time). That was fine, so we'll see what's going on tomorrow afternoon. Congratulations to our Ryan for getting the writing award again. Very proud of our Colorado kid, even though he asked me on the phone, "Grandma, did you ever fart and blame someone else?"

THURSDAY, OCTOBER 25, 2007

Went to gastroenterologist today to check the J-tube. All is in order. He probably leaked so much the other night because there is so much fluid in his stomach. They are setting up an out-patient procedure where they remove some of the liquid from his stomach to make him more comfortable. Too bad they can't do the same thing for his feet and legs. So Big Foot will have to wait until they start acting like normal limbs again. From the doctor, we went to Sam's Club to pick up some meds. While there, Gerry saw the Wolfgang Puck griddle/grill and fell in love with the new-fangled cooking device. We are now the proud owners of said grill. Oy!

Friday, October 26, 2007

Quite a weather change. From beautiful and in the
70's to raining and in the 40's. I asked Gerry what he
wanted for lunch and he requested scrambled eggs
with salsa topping. And he ate every bit! Grumpy is
doing pretty well except for the Big Feet. Poor guy can't
lift them onto the bed without help. That's where Nurse
Ratched comes in handy. Wish the damn swelling
would go down already!

Saturday, October 27, 2007

Rainy, rainy day. Ronni came out for overnight visit
while Eric and Scott sat in the pouring rain watching
Rutgers lose (badly) to West Virginia. We screamed at
the TV set, but it didn't help. Gerry ordered hot dogs on
his new Wolfgang Puck toy, and the food was delicious!
Andrea just finished a school project: a clay depiction
of the Western (Wailing) Wall in Israel. This is the wall
where visitors put little pieces of paper into the cracks,
praying for someone or something. Nicole told her to
put a piece of paper in her project saying "I'm praying
for an A." Don't think she's taking this sisterly advice.
Ryan is getting ready for Halloween. He wants to be a
gangster and put the costume together all by himself.
Amy says he looks more like the Blues Brothers.

Great day today. Sherry and Jim came to visit, bringing
a DVD of our great nephew Michael's Bar Mitzvah.
Next best thing to being there. Michael is the son of
Adam (Sherry's brother) and Jill (Amy's friend from
Junior High). Since Amy introduced them, I guess
she can add matchmaker to her resume. Also have to
mention Michael's little sister, Jenna, or Stanley the
Grandpa would never forgive me.

Grumpy got an early Chanukah present from his
kids: an iPod Nano that plays 2000 songs, plus shows,
pictures and movies. He's learning how to use it for
his next chemo date. In addition, they gave him a web
cam that allows him to see and talk to the person on
the other end. They did this because Gerry and his
big brother Stan have not been able to get together in
person. Looks like a little alien on top of the computer
screen. Ain't technology great? Since our boy doesn't
get out that often, he loves communicating by web
cam and phone. The calls from Stanley and Joel really
cheer him up! Gerry has ordered Chinese food for
tonight. Guess he's feeling better.

MONDAY, OCTOBER 29, 2007

It took three calls to the doctor's office, but we finally
got a call back on Gerry's procedure-to-be. It is called
paracentesis and will take place Thursday. Susi and
Andrea are preparing a Rachel Ray dinner tonight.
Gerry watches the cooking shows and lets us know
what looks good to him...even though most food tastes
like tin since he started the new chemo. Nicole had
a mid term (did well) and then donated blood. Why?
Because she got a free t-shirt and a purple bandage.

TUESDAY, OCTOBER 30, 2007

Had our chemo date today and the platelet dance is
working. The count was way up again and Gerry was
able to get his third chemo in a row. He brought his
new iPod and all of a sudden, a loud voice in the key of
OFF started singing, "Oo oo oo oo oooo you've got that
lovin' feeling." The PA came into the room asked what
that song was. Gerry told her. She asked who sang it.
He told her: The Righteous Brothers. She said, "Why
don't you just let them sing it?" Just kidding. They
love him there!

WEDNESDAY, OCTOBER 31, 2007

Funny thing happened while I was speaking to my brother Joel last night. He said, "The house is shaking. Wow! It's an earthquake!" No damage to the house, just to the nervous system. Ryan put on his gangster costume for trick and treating. A suit, shirt and tie and large sunglasses. At the last minute, he didn't like the sunglasses, so he took them off, looked in the mirror, and said, "I'm going as a businessman." Gerry and Nicole were using the PC cameras today and could see each other while speaking on regular phones. Have to figure out how to coordinate sound and picture. Oh, to be computer savvy!

THURSDAY, NOVEMBER 1, 2007

Today was paracentesis day. Got up at 6 A.M. so Gerry could have his breakfast-in-a-tube before 7 A.M. You have to fast 4 hours before procedure. Got to hospital at 9:30 for blood work and no one was at the reception desk. Went back a few minutes later and the lady in charge appeared. I gave her Gerry's name and she said she'd get back to us. At 9:50 I went back to same lady and told her procedure was scheduled for 11 A.M. Shouldn't they be taking his blood? She told me we should have been there at 9:30. I smiled nicely (gritting my teeth) and told her we were there...she wasn't. She finally got us an outpatient room and they started Grumpy on an IV and took blood. About 11:45 we went to radiology department where he was to get an ultrasound while they searched for the fluid in his abdomen. They sent me back to his room and told me to wait. They would notify me when procedure was done. I was in the room about fifteen minutes when the nurse came in and said they didn't do the procedure. There wasn't enough fluid to warrant it. So the poor guy had to go through all that crap for nothing! Guess it was good in a way. Maybe the swelling in his belly is going down. Problem is, it's going down into Big Foot's legs. He had a snack there and Susi gave him a nice lunch when we came home. He is resting now after watching Rachel Ray's 30-minute-meal cooking show. What optimism!

Friday, November 2, 2007

Got a call from our long-time camping friends, Al and Alice. They asked if we were up to company this afternoon and we said YES! To reward them for their hour drive, I served up some Irish coffee (a la Buena Vista in San Francisco). Gerry had one, also...and he's still smiling. In fact he is overjoyed! It didn't taste like tin.

Saturday, November 3, 2007

Our Scott is 18 today. Tried to call to wish him a happy birthday, but there was no answer. We left him a singing message and he called back to say he and Ronni were at the Motor Vehicle Bureau. Now that he's 18, he gets his regular driver's license! Gerry was all set to watch the Rutgers game today, but they can only watch our team in Arizona, New Mexico, Oregon and Southern California. Makes perfect sense! But he has enough football to keep him busy all weekend. The patient finally had some unwanted results from the newest chemo. He ran like the Energizer bunny this morning, but is fine now. Even talking about what's for dinner! That's my boy!

SUNDAY, NOVEMBER 4, 2007

We have this new alarm clock that flashes the time on the ceiling. Pretty neat! At 2 A.M. we both woke up to see if the time would change automatically (fall ahead/spring back time). It didn't change. Woke up again at 5 A.M. and it worked! The little things that make you happy. Gerry had trouble swallowing his pills a few days ago. He could swallow soft foods, but the pills gave him a problem. Yesterday I told him I'd give him two soft-boiled eggs. Easier said than done. Put the eggs in the water, waited for water to boil and set timer for three minutes. Evidently, the water wasn't boiled enough, because when I cracked the eggs open, there were two yolks floating in water. To salvage this gourmet dish, I put the eggs in the microwave, and ended up with two eggs floating in rubber. So last night I ordered an electric egg boiler/poacher. How can Nurse Ratched go wrong with such an up-to-date, fancy gadget?

Monday, November 5, 2007

Gerry wasn't feeling too well, so we went to the doctor
a day early. She is sending him for a thoracentesis
tomorrow, taking liquid out of his lungs. She'll start
next round of chemo Thursday of this week. He's still
watching cooking shows even though he isn't able to
eat much lately. Always the optimist! Got RX for
liquid pain meds, and will pick them up tomorrow.
In the meantime, percocet crushed in apple sauce
does the trick. Amy and Ryan may come in for
Thanksgiving week. Wouldn't that be great medicine?
The patient is looking forward to Monday night
football. Nurse Ratched isn't, but what the hell.
Whatever makes him happy!

Tuesday, November 6, 2007

Today was thorocentesis day. Got to hospital at 8 A.M.,
with Ronni as assistant to Nurse Ratched. Got Gerry
settled, and they took him down for this procedure
(just like last week). But this time it worked. They
brought him back to his room about 45 minutes later,
and told us they extracted about 1-1/2 liters of fluid
from his lungs. Stayed in the hospital till about 12:45
and then went to pick up his Zofran (for nausea). He
has to take this the day before, day of and day after
chemo. Also picked up liquid morphine for pain. Right
now the patient is fast asleep in lala land. Today

was a phenomenal day for communicating via Web Cam. First we saw brother Stanley in Lynchburg, Va. Later on we were contacted by Amy and Ryan in Colorado. While they were on, niece Naomi joined us from San Francisco, and we got to see Edwin, Cameron and Jackson. While we were on, Naomi's brother, our nephew Simeon, joined in from Ashland, OR. We looked at each other while speaking into our telephones. Have to figure out how to get the sound to work, but this was such a treat!

WEDNESDAY, NOVEMBER 7, 2007

Nurse Ratched strikes again! After Gerry had his meds this morning, he sat in his electric chair. I put his support stockings on, arranged a pillow behind his back and asked him if he needed a blanket. He said yes, so I took a pretty afghan, and toreador style, swung it onto the patient with a flourish. Then I heard, "OUCH!" Seems I swung it a little too hard and hit him in the chest where the fluid was removed yesterday. Oops! Good thing he had his pain meds first! The patient is feeling a little better today. He ate two soft-boiled eggs, Jello and whipped cream. Tomorrow is chemo day.

Thursday, November 8, 2007

Had our chemo date, and when we were through, Gerry decided he wanted KFC for dinner. He saw an ad for triple chicken strips with dipping sauce, etc. So we stopped and bought this item plus a large bucket of whatever, and when we got home, he couldn't wait for dinner. So he ate one of the chicken strips for lunch and had the rest of the finger-lickin'-chicken at dinner time with no swallowing problems. Right now the patient is watching some cooking shows with Susi. They're planning a big Thanksgiving feast and want to find some very special recipes.

Friday, November 9, 2007

It's a cold and rainy day, but that doesn't dampen Grumpy's interest in cooking shows. Loves to watch what he hopes to be able to eat any day now. We're so different. Gerry Boy lives to eat and I eat to live. So far he has been able to swallow some apple juice without gagging, and that's a good sign. I think the new liquid pain meds are helping to control his discomfort. He weighed himself today, and since they removed all that fluid the other day, he lost about 14 pounds. The support hose have also helped reduce the fluid in his legs. Looking forward to the Michelsons visiting this weekend and Amy and Ryan flying in a week from tomorrow. Our college girl came home last night and Nicole and Andrea entertained "Dewald" with their stories (when Susi baby-sat last year, her little charge, Rachel, used to call him "Dewald". She also called herself "Wachel."). Susi did some major shopping today, getting ready for Thanksgiving. Matt is hoping to work only a 6-day week and stay home this Sunday. What a great family we have – near and far. Our daughters have always been close to their poppy and very special. The sons-in-law have also stepped up to the plate. Matt visits with Gerry every night when he comes home from work, before ever going upstairs for dinner. Mark calls him a few times a week from his cell phone en route from work to home, and they have great, very positive conversations. Carl speaks to him weekly, also with upbeat talk, and regrets not joining us for Thanksgiving.

Saturday, November 10, 2007

Woke up this morning to see snow covering the lawns. Quite a surprise! By afternoon, it all melted. The Michelsons came out for an overnight visit and Gerry just loves the company. Ronni's friend Ellen came out this afternoon (she's like our fourth daughter), and we're having a wonderful day. Got an e-mail from Amazon telling me the electric egg cooker/poacher has been delayed in manufacturing. Not ready for shipment until mid-January. The gods don't want me to make good boiled eggs, evidently. So I cancelled the order, and will go looking in the stores. Tonight we're having ziti marinara, garlic bread and Caesar salad for dinner. I think the patient will not have any problems with the ziti.

SUNDAY, NOVEMBER 11, 2007

Gerry is happy with football all day. I'm happy watching him happy. Just had one of my famous Irish coffees, so the football is much more enjoyable. Matt's sister Liz, from Tennessee, e-mailed to tell me she just ordered an egg boiler/poacher. It will be so great to have eggs that are edible. What a grand gesture! The patient is looking very happy with his liquid morphine. The boys went back to college today. Nicole goes back tomorrow, and come Saturday, Amy and Ryan arrive. Full house for Thanksgiving. The whole gang (except for Carl, who can't get away) will be here. Yeah!

MONDAY, NOVEMBER 12, 2007

Cold and dreary day. Grumpy was a little grumpy today. He does much better when it's sunny and bright. The liquid pain med is making him one happy boy, though. He spent today reading, sleeping and answering my questions in sign language and grunts — just to be funny. Even if the patient can't eat everything, food is still important to him. Don't know what he likes more. Football or Food Network!

Tuesday, November 13, 2007

Pretty quiet day today. Gerry was a little "loopy" from the pain meds, so I went to Sam's Club by myself and came back with all kinds of goodies, including Shrek III. Watched it this afternoon. Funny movie, especially for adults who have never grown up. Tomorrow is rheumatology day, and I'm hoping he shoots me in the knee. The patient is deciding if he wants dinner on a plate or in the tube. By the way, Liz's egg cooker arrived today. Can't wait to make un-screwed-up boiled eggs. Even comes with a recipe for Eggs Benedict!

Wednesday, November 14, 2007

It is a dark and dreary day...rain coming in, but who cares? I got shot in the knee. Whoopee! I'll be limp-free for 2-3 days. Grumpster didn't feel like going out today, so he stayed home with Susi to watch (what else?) cooking shows. We have cut back on the liquid morphine a bit. Instead of every 3 hours, he's going to try every 5 hours. Of course, if he needs it sooner, he'll get it. The morphine makes him sleepy and loopy (or as Ronni says – disoriented.) He doesn't like that feeling, and neither does Nurse Ratched. He was acting like a few of the dwarfs: Grumpy, Dopey, Sleepy and Happy. Right now we're watching HGTV. I can take just so much of cooking shows.

Thursday, November 15, 2007

Went on our chemo date today, driving through a downpour. But the platelet count was up. Guess platelet dance worked! Now we have to do a dance for the chemo to work. Will try chicken soup with matzo balls tonight. Hope Gerry can have more than Ensure for dinner. Spoke to Naomi in San Francisco, and she said she made chicken soup for the boys when they had colds. Jackson, the two-year-old, said,"Mom, the chicken soup don't work!" Let's hope I have better luck.

Friday, November 16, 2007

Grumpy agreed with Jackson last night. The chicken soup didn't work. After the chemo, everything tastes like tin. Because he's having trouble swallowing, Ronni suggested we get all his meds in liquid form. Picked them all up today, and for dinner the patient had Ensure and all the yucky meds right down the tube. Sherry and Jim are coming tomorrow for the day, and Amy and Ryan arrive tomorrow night. Matt will pick them up at Newark Airport on the way home from work. Looking forward to all the company.

Saturday, November 17, 2007

Sherry and Jim came for a few hours. Sherry and Gerry watched football and yelled at the TV set. Jim and I had a more civilized afternoon, drinking Irish Coffee. Gerry decided that Irish Coffee sounded good, so I made him one and he downed ¾ of it. Way to go, Gerry! Sherry and Jim have been such steadfast, devoted visitors. They pick up Gerry's spirits with every visit, and there have been plenty of visits. We're watching Amy's flight on the PC. Right now they're over the Great Lakes and should be arriving a little after 6 P.M. The patient did very well with all the meds down the tube. Nurse Ratched was superb. Didn't spill a drop on him!

Sunday, November 18, 2007

Amy and Ryan arrived last night, and the first thing Amy said when she saw Gerry was, "Gee, you don't look as bad as I thought you would!" Exciting day in Pine Island. Nicole went to recycling with Matt. Andrea jumped in the leaves with Ryan. Amy's school pal, Sue, came to visit and brought delicious cheesecake. The patient was only able to eat two bites. Being Sunday, it's football day for Gerry and Amy. Amy is keeping a close watch on the teams she picked in her office football pool. So far, she has one right! Gerry spent a good deal of time sleeping through the games, and here I am — watching what I don't want to watch so I can keep him company when he wakes up.

Monday, November 19, 2007

Woke up this morning to find the lawn covered with
at least two inches of snow. Got a little concerned
because Susi and I had a doctor's appointment in White
Plains...a good 1-1/2 hour trip. But the roads were
perfectly fine, and as we neared the Tappan Zee Bridge,
all traces of snow disappeared. Ronni came out this
morning, and she, Amy and Ryan kept Gerry company.
Got home at 5:45 and all was well. Gerry got a few
phone calls from a few of his friends, and that really
lifted his spirits.

Tuesday, November 20, 2007

What a nice day. Claire (my college roommate) and
Marty came out to visit and brought dinner...from
soup to dessert and everything in-between. Don't
think my Gerry Boy will be able to eat it, but we'll all
enjoy the scrumptious food. The weather is so foggy,
they decided to leave early before they could join us for
the feast. Ryan met them, and he heard so much about
them, he thought ClaireandMarty was one word. Nicole
comes home for the holiday weekend. Scotty is making
Grumpy's favorite pumpkin bread and the patient
hopes he can eat a little of it. Eric is continuing his
job interviews. Can't believe he graduates this coming
Spring! Since we started the liquid meds, Gerry

doesn't have to worry about swallowing. He spends a good deal of time sleeping. That morphine really does a number on you! When Andrea comes home from school and starts singing, he wakes up with a big grin! Going to eat an early dinner tonight so we can watch one of Gerry's favorite TV shows together with him: Charlie Brown's Thanksgiving.

WEDNESDAY, NOVEMBER 21, 2007

We had our chemo date today. Gerry looked much better after the treatment than when he came in for it. Loved Claire and Marty's dinner last night and had enough left over for tonight. Susi's friend, Creslyn, brought over ice cream cake for dessert, Yum! Got a package from Sherry and Jim today containing a heated massage pad for cars and chairs. It was so thoughtful, but there was one problem. You can't get heat without a massage, and it was too bumpy for the boy. And yes, they're getting the present back with regrets. Right now the kids are upstairs making Thanksgiving decorations for tomorrow.

THURSDAY, NOVEMBER 22, 2007

The gang's all here (except Carl, spending the holiday with his family in Colorado). The big bird is in the oven (not to be confused with Big Bird on Sesame Street). Eric, Scott and Ryan had a little football game going in the backyard. The girls played Guitar Hero with Ryan, and he's quite the player. He can beat you standing upside down and backwards. Gerry is mostly sleeping today. The meds really knock him out. Funny though, he wakes up every time Green Bay scores a touchdown. Had a wonderful dinner and Gerry enjoyed watching everyone else eat. Loves being surrounded by family! And Andrea brought her plate over to the couch to keep Grumpy company!

Friday, November 23, 2007

What a lazy morning. Too much food last night. Reminded me of the time we decided to do Thanksgiving dinner sans turkey. We made a Mongolian Fire Pot instead. Took hours to prepare and hours to eat, and there were no leftovers. So the next day I bought a turkey, cooked it, and everyone went home with care packages. Last night we watched "Mr. and Mrs. Smith." Brad and Angelina are beautiful, but where was the script? Tonight we're going for "Ice Age Meltdown II." Tonight we also used the Web Cam and saw relatives from California to Virginia, but we still haven't been able to figure out the sound. We write messages to each other. Oh, to be computer literate!

Saturday, November 24, 2007

Cold day today, but Andrea and Ryan managed to catch some time outdoors. We stayed inside with Gerry. First it was football, then a movie called "Deja Vu." Gerry and Ronni liked it. The rest of us are shaking our heads and saying, "What happened?" So far the patient has been able to eat canned pears and peaches and has had a little decaf coffee. We are thrilled to see him consume anything!

Sunday, November 25, 2007

Was a good night last night. Grumpy slept through for the first time in months. That means Nurse Ratched also had a great sleep. Gerry had his first boiled egg in a few weeks (thanks, Liz). He's still eating the canned pears and peaches every day, but everything else is down the tube. Today is Gerry's dream day. Football from noon until whenever. Mark and the boys left yesterday. Mark continues to call Gerry several times a week for "zen time," and the talks really help. Ronni left this morning, Nicole goes back to school tomorrow morning, and Amy and Ryan leave tomorrow afternoon. Then we start counting the days till they return in December.

Monday, November 26, 2007

Amy and Ryan were picked up by limo at 2 P.M. and arrived at Newark Airport with plenty of time to spare. They called from Nathan's, where they were enjoying a snack, and then Ryan had time to buy some NY souvenirs. House is mighty quiet without the mob. Susi, Gerry and I watched another movie "Hostage," with Bruce Willis. This time we picked a good one. Gerry didn't even fall asleep! Today the patient had a bowl of fruit and yogurt and was able to eat it all!

TUESDAY, NOVEMBER 27, 2007

Went to oncologist today. On the way, I said to Grumpy,
"I love you!" He looked at me and said, "I love you,
too, but I'd love you more if you stopped hitting the
bumps!" A real Romeo. Doctor seems to think he's
doing pretty well on the new chemo. She's increasing
the dose a little, and after the third round, they'll take
more pictures. In the meantime, the tired patient is
tired for a reason. His hemoglobin count is very low.
So Thursday we have a transfusion date, when he gets 2
units of blood. That'll make him perky!

WEDNESDAY, NOVEMBER 28, 2007

Went to hospital today to get Gerry's blood cross-
checked for tomorrow's transfusion. He is so looking
forward to feeling peppy again. Today we had a great
visit from dear friends Carol and Irwin. Loved the
company and also loved the care package they brought:
tonight's dinner. If Carol wasn't anxious about driving
at night, they would have joined us. That's what friends
are for. Susi and Andrea went Chanukah shopping
after school today. Nicole takes a bus into White Plains
from school, and does her shopping there. Looking
forward to the holidays!

Thursday, November 29, 2007

Had our "vampire" date today. Gerry got 2 units of blood and what a difference! Took him into Tucker Center in a wheel chair, and seven hours later he walked out! He just had his dinner-in-a-tube, but is still talking about what he can really eat tomorrow. May try some tilapia in wine and mushroom sauce. Tonight we watch Rutgers football. It's one of the few football games I enjoy watching. Hoping to see Eric and Scotty in the stands, but so far no luck. Seems that thousands of people all show up in red shirts!

Friday, November 30. 2007

Today was our go-to-podiatrist date. Gerry was a bit tired. Even though yesterday's transfusion left him with "perky" blood, the patient wasn't feeling very perky. Today is Eric's last day as an underage kid. Tomorrow he's a drinking man, and we hear his friends are taking him out to a bar at midnight to make it official. Can't believe he's 21! Susi and the girls wrapped a bunch of Chanukah gifts last night, and the piano became the Chanukah center. Looks so pretty decorated with gorgeous gift-wrapped stuff. Guess I'll make latkes tomorrow!

Gerry is having a pretty good day today, and he's
looking forward to friggin' football all day and night.
One happy guy! He did eat a little pork roast last night,
and that made us all very happy. Got a call from Amy
last night to tell us that Carl and Ryan were in a car
accident. Some bozo hit Carl with such force, the
air bag popped. Ryan was in the back seat, but got a
bloody lip, sore head, etc. Both went to the hospital
to be checked out, and they'll be fine (eventually...
they got quite a jolt). Amy asked Ryan what he wanted
for a special gift and he mentioned something that
costs about $120. Amy said to think of something for
about twenty bucks, and he said, "But Mom, it was a
car accident!" That ploy didn't work! I did something
stupid yesterday. Went to drugstore and was wearing
my sunglasses. I put them on top of my head, and
when I got back to the car, I couldn't find them...
until I realized where I put them. When I went to the
next store, I put them in my pocket for safe-keeping.
Finished shopping, got back in the car and heard a
strange noise. You see, the jacket was long, the pocket
was low, and I sat on my glasses, breaking the ear
piece off. Lenscrafter, here I come! Eric is 21 today
and recovering from his night out with friends last
evening. Tonight we'll watch "Hairspray" upstairs
while the Grumpster watches football downstairs.

SUNDAY, DECEMBER 2, 2007

Woke up to promised snow. Tonight they predict ice, but right now there is enough snow for Matt to run circles around the house on his snowmobile. One happy fellow! Another happy fellow is Gerry, who's feeling pretty good today. He's watching one football game after another, working on paperwork at his desk and drinking coffee. Ryan and Carl are both doing pretty well after the accident, but will go to doctor tomorrow for checkup, to make sure all systems are go.

MONDAY, DECEMBER 3, 2007

Watched pictures on TV of terrible wind damage in the New York area. Looked out the window and said, "What wind?" So far, we've been lucky. Hope weather is good tomorrow for our chemo date. Grumpy had his usual yogurt and fruit for lunch, but he didn't do too well with the tilapia last night. Too chewy. The consistency of the food can bother him. Nicole has the same problem because of the MHE disorder. Tonight we'll try cup-a-soup.

Tuesday, December 4, 2007

Chemo date started with freezing wind and 29 degrees temperature. We blew into the doctor's office, and everything was great after that. Platelet count was up and the doc upped his new chemo recipe (taxitere). For the past two days Gerry has been feeling stronger. Guess the transfusion finally kicked in. Did not need a walker or a cane today, and he sang off-key to Brooks and Dunne during chemo. Patient has a sinus infection, so we stopped at drug store on way home to get a liquid antibiotic — which goes right down the tube. Nicole is 19 today, and Matt will stop by at her dorm to take her to dinner. First Chanukah candle tonight.

Wednesday, December 5, 2007

So it snowed all day today. Luckily, the roads are clear. Had to go out and buy ingredients for the potato pancakes. What's Chanukah without latkes? Will make them when Nicole comes home, and Gerry may try to eat some. Think the antibiotic is starting to kick in. Patient is not coughing as much. Ordered a new web cam which arrived today. As soon as Susi gets in touch with Gerry's brother Stan, he'll talk her through the installation. I'm too chicken to tackle it. Maybe now we'll be able to see each other and speak!!!!

THURSDAY, DECEMBER 6, 2007

Gerry had another good day. Had cup-a-soup for lunch (sure beats food down the tube). With Stanley's help, Susi set up our new web cam. So exciting to be able to see and speak to each other in distant places. The brothers were thrilled to have a virtual meeting.

FRIDAY, DECEMBER 7, 2007

Surprise! It snowed again today! Only one in the house who loves the white stuff is Matt. Ronni came out late this afternoon and only had bad road conditions the last few miles to our house. Eric and Scott are planning to come out tomorrow, weather permitting. This afternoon we watched the movie "Waitress." What a wonderful film! The patient is having a pretty good day, but the sinuses haven't cleared up completely, so he could be happier. But he's still feeling stronger than he did last week. Time for a chemo dance.

SATURDAY, DECEMBER 8, 2007

Pretty cloudy, crummy day again. Matt went to work, but came home at 4:30 this afternoon. Half a day for him. Jim and Sherry came out for a visit, and Eric and Scott arrived a few minutes later. I made latkes for lunch and we had a great time. Gerry is not having a great day because of the bad weather coming in tomorrow. Arthritis is bothering him more than the cancer! Ronni bought "Oceans 13" today and we may watch it later. Right now, Gerry Boy is watching basketball. Tomorrow it's football again. What a loyal sports fan. We celebrated Chanukah tonight, and the girls gave Gerry a very funny, sick present: a T-shirt from the musical "Spamalot" with following saying on front, "I'm Not Dead Yet." Knowing our warped sense of humor, some of you may laugh and some may turn green. Mark gave Gerry a Rutgers shirt, so we took pix of him wearing both additions to his wardrobe.

SUNDAY, DECEMBER 9, 2007

With the forecast of rain turning to snow or ice later, Ronni and the boys left at noon. Matt, Susi and Andrea drove Nicole back to college a day early, so she wouldn't miss her finals. The patient is a little less achy today, but very tired from the combo of antibiotics, liquid morphine and cough medicine. But it's football day... all day... so Gerry is a very happy guy. And he's wearing his Rutgers shirt while screaming at the television.

MONDAY, DECEMBER 10, 2007

Grumpy is feeling a little shaky on his legs these past few days, so he's boogying around with his walker. He's wondering if the extra chemo he got last week may have something to do with it, so we'll check it out on our chemo date tomorrow. Spent the afternoon watching past episodes of "The Shield" with Susi. Addicted to this sicko series. Then Ry Guy got an award in his 4th grade class today for having a 3.5 GPA. No school here today because of the ice, so Andrea redecorated her room. Haven't seen it yet, but I know it's incredible.

Went to our chemo date today, but Gerry did not get chemo. He wanted to speak to the doctor, because he's been feeling very weak for the past week. She decided to wait a week to give his system a chance to get some of the "poison" out. Gerry wore his "Spamalot" shirt to the office today that says "I'm Not Dead Yet." The doctor suggested that a Hospice nurse visit twice a week for a few weeks to give us a hand on how to help the patient (getting up from chair, bed, etc.). When Gerry heard the word Hospice, he said, "Does that mean I have to change my shirt?" The doctor said NO!!! What a brave guy. And what a sense of humor. Gotta love him!

The rep from Hospice came this morning to go over all the details. We'll have nurse and aide available... as well as a social worker. I told her we already had a social worker in the family (Ronni). She said that you need an outsider, who will be available once a month or more, if requested. I told her about my experience with a social worker in Florida. Right after my breast cancer surgery she came in and said that they were having a gathering in a park in a few weeks. We would be given balloons and we could fly them up in the air. Goodbye- to-cancer symbolism. I told her to get lost (in polite words). One of the benefits of

Hospice, besides the wonderful people, is that they supply Ensure, bandages, paper tape, etc. etc. We were spending a fortune on that stuff. Gotta look on the bright side of life (another song from "Spamalot"). The nurse is calling us tomorrow morning to set up an appointment, but there is a major snow storm expected, so we may have to wait till next week. Not to worry. Nurse Ratched has it covered (but with Hospice being in the picture now, am I being naïve?). Susi did a major shopping today, getting ready for the winter wonderland. Matt will bring Nicole home tonight so she's not stuck in school all weekend. The only one happy about forthcoming storm is Matt. He can ride his snowmobile.

Thursday, December 13, 2007

Not a good day today. Bad snow storm. More than six inches right now and still coming down. Because of the storm, Hospice nurse called to say she couldn't come this morning. And of all days, Gerry wasn't feeling well. Couldn't breathe when he lay down and couldn't sit up without difficulty. Susi and I were sitting with him on the side of the bed and all of a sudden his eyes rolled back and he seemed to be in a different place. We started screaming at him, and he snapped out of the state he was in and started responding. Scared the hell out of us. We called Hospice and they sent over oxygen. As soon as he started getting the extra oxygen, his breathing was much better. He stopped wheezing and was very comfortable. He's been in a deep sleep all day and doesn't appear to be in any pain or discomfort. The oxygen contraption is a large gizmo that we had to make room for. The delivery man told us he delivered another contraption during this morning's snow storm and the lady of the house refused it. Didn't go with her home décor. Go figure! Hospice people have been calling all day to walk us through all our questions. Never thought we'd reach this stage so soon!

Friday, December 14, 2007

As we enter a new phase of our journey, we ask everyone to send loving vibes to Grumpy. He took a turn for the worse, and Hospice delivered a hospital bed today to make him more comfortable. Amy and Ryan were supposed to come in next Friday, but we changed the tickets and they're arriving tomorrow. Ronni, Mark and the boys came out today, and he's surrounded by a bunch of loving kids and grandkids (not to mention Nurse Ratched). He's not in pain, resting very comfortably and is one sweet, loving, wonderful patient.

Gerry is sleeping most of the afternoon, but this morning he was in fine humor. Mark told him his color was good and his fingernail color was good. Gerry replied, "If my color is so good, so all this fuss is about nothing?" He then gave Eric and Scott some special jewelry, and told them he didn't have many valuables, but it was important they have this. He said the only valuable he wasn't giving away was Audrey. Ronni was helping me turn the patient in the hospital bed and he said, "You're too slow. You're not professionals." Guess he's used to the Hospice expertise. Cousin Bobbie called and asked if he could talk. He said, "Sure. I do funny one-liners." And then he said that when Amy arrives today, she's going to walk in and say, "Gee you look better than I thought you would." Matt is picking them up this afternoon. When people call, he actually gets on the phone, perks up and speaks to each caller for a short time. Joel and Diane called from California and we heard a genuine belly laugh coming from the patient. Jim and Sherry wanted to know how he was feeling. Gerry said, "I'm feeling. As long as I'm feeling, I guess I'm fine." Cousin Harriet called from Florida, and he said "I love Harriet!" Gerry told Ronni to thank Mark for the hospital bed. She told him that Mark did a lot to help him, but the bed was from Hospice. Susi and the girls went shopping for the whole gang who will be coming and going this week. Got Amy's Freihoffer cookies, so she'll be happy. Can't get them in Colorado.

Gerry is holding his own. Had a restful night and good morning, until I fed him the Ensure through the tube...then Grumpy became Leaky. Everything started pouring out of the tube opening for an hour or so. We were running for towels and bandages and Kleenex and anything to stop the flow. Called the Hospice nurse, who came over in this horrible weather, cleaned the boy up and made him more comfortable. No more Ensure is the moral of this story. When Amy and Ryan arrived last night, Amy came into the room and said, "Hey, Dad, you don't look as good as I thought you would." Gerry said, "It's good to see you here." Amy said, "It's good to see YOU here, too." This morning Gerry was thirsty. We gave him sponges on a stick, dipped in water. While he was sucking on the sponge, Amy walked in drinking a frappacino. He said, "I'm the one who's thirsty, and you're drinking a frappacino!!" Sherry and Jim came over from South Jersey (3-hour trip each way). They left early because of the weather. Gerry wanted to know why they were leaving so soon. They said it was because it was so bad outside. Gerry told them it was pretty nice inside. Maybe they should stay! Matt took Ryan out for a snowmobile ride before the sleet and rain started. The boy had a blast. Now Ryan is playing Guitar Hero with his cousins. The patient is sleeping through the football game. Must really be tired. This afternoon he was able to speak to his Virginia kin, Maryland kin, etc. And all the caregivers enjoyed the desserts that Creslyn brought over last night!

<h2 style="text-align:center">Monday, December 17, 2007</h2>

Hospice nurse just left. She said Gerry looked a little better than when she saw him a few days ago. Got him all comfortable, but he's having trouble with the feeding tube. We tried just water and liquid meds and he became leaky again. Tomorrow she may try to replace the tube, per conversation with the doctor who inserted it. Gerry is very comfortable right now and that's what counts!

<h2 style="text-align:center">Tuesday, December 18, 2007</h2>

Not a good day for Grumpy. His breathing was very heavy and strained during the night. The patient slept, but Nurse Ratched was up all night watching him. We called Hospice at 6 A.M. and a nurse showed up at 7 to make him comfortable. Later in the morning, our Hospice RN, Joanne, came along with a wonderful practical nurse called Marty. They helped raise his comfort level and told us to call at any time if we need them. We mentioned to Joanne that Gerry's eyes looked a little strange. She said that he was nearing the end and was seeing something beyond. She also said that he may be seeing his parents. We screamed in unison, "Not his mother!"

Gerry is surrounded by his girls, grandson Ryan and granddaughter Andrea. Nicole, Eric and Scott keep calling from college, but they have finals this week, and promised their grandpa they'd do well for him. But they're here in spirit. Carl wrote Gerry a beautiful letter that Amy read to him, and Carl's music CD is playing in the bedroom – so beautiful and so soothing. The phone just rang, and Gerry woke up long enough to say, "I can't talk now." He then whispered to me that he was getting so disgusted with the condition he was in. I told him that he was so brave and so loved, but he could let go. We would all be fine and he needn't worry. The phone call was from old friends in Florida and Susi took the call in the living room. She was so busy consoling them, she was not in the room for Gerry's final moments.

And suddenly, our cosmic journey has come to an end. My darling Gerry passed away this evening and we still can't believe it. He was so uncomfortable all day, and toward evening we turned him on his side. He had a sudden surge of energy and reached out and hugged me, stared at me intently, and then stared into an unknown space. We hugged each other and he died in my arms. In fact, his passing was so peaceful, we didn't realize he had transitioned until the Hospice nurse came in, took out her stethoscope and said, "He's gone." Amy and I were still in denial, saying things like he's breathing much better, no more gasping for breath. Then Ronni realized what just happened and said, "Daddy, when I told you it was O.K. to let go, I didn't really mean it!"

He was such an incredible human being, full of love and joy and wisdom and generosity. Knowing that he's no longer in pain makes it much easier for all of us. We still feel his presence everywhere in the house, and most importantly, he's in all of our hearts forever.

The Aftershock

Shock is a very good thing. You go through everyday activities by rote, still not comprehending what just happened. Gerry is not here physically, but we all feel his spirit, and are happy that his suffering is over. He always said, "It is what it is," and that's a sobering comment.

Funeral Planning

We had pre-planned our final arrangements, so at least we didn't have to make decisions when we were in no position to make decisions. Yes, shock was still propelling us on. We settled on Friday morning, December 21, and arranged for food to be picked up that morning for the group expected back after the services. Gerry's main wish was for donations to be made to the MHE Coalition. MHE is a painful bone disorder that our granddaughter Nicole lives with on a daily basis. We let his wish be known and contributions started pouring in. How proud our Grumpy would have been. We were so busy planning, we forgot to eat today. Luckily, friends Noreen and Tina sent over a beautiful spread and we discovered we were hungry.

Hours Before the Funeral

We were up at the crack of dawn preparing for our
Grumpy farewell. Last night Susi and the girls
prepared 2 poster boards with wonderful pictures of
our Gerry boy, which will be on display
at the services. Something strange happened last
night. I touched Gerry's side of the bed and it was
warm. I checked to see if I put on his electric blanket
switch by mistake, but it was off. Guess he was visiting.
It still seems surreal, but something we'll have to
get used to…in time. Friend Creslyn volunteered to
come over to our house to prepare all the food for the
after-funeral gathering. There is one certainty in life.
Whether it's a celebration or a funeral, you have to eat!

The Funeral

A long day, but a beautiful day. The Purta Funeral
Home was so caring, and our Grumpy looked so
peaceful (even happy), that it lifted a big load from our
hearts. Rabbi Stemler, who conducted the service, was
so warm and sincere, it was hard to believe we never
met him before today. He has since called our home
on a regular basis, checking in on the family. Gerry
had so many loving friends and family. Even those
who were not there in person, were there in spirit.

Many of us spoke at the service: Ronni first, then Mark, then Amy, then Carl, then Susi, then Sherry, and finally Nurse Ratched...who even sang a few lines to end her eulogy. What's a Feldman gathering without a song? I just sang a parody of "Send in the Clowns" (with apologies to Sondheim).

"Isn't it rich? Are we a pair? Me with my head in the clouds. I'll find you up there. Where are the clouds? Send in the clouds. I'll find you somewhere."

THREE MILES TO THE CEMETERY

There was a crowd at the service, including the Hospice nurse and social worker, who only knew Gerry a few days, but felt the love in the family. Then on to the cemetery. Our three sons-in-law, 3 grandsons and nephew Jim were pallbearers. Yes, Ryan helped carry Grumpy to his final resting place. After a brief service, we all went back to our house to visit with our wonderful family and friends, and, of course, to eat. We bought too much food, but there's always tomorrow, and tomorrow, and...

Celebrating Grumpy

When most of the folks left, the few remaining decided to celebrate Gerry with music: Carl at the piano; Kenny, Eric. Ronni, Susi and Sharon on guitars; Mark on the harmonica; Sharon, Ronni, Amy, Susi and myself doing vocals; Scott and Ryan in the rhythm section. It was a musical relief from the last 8 months. We're still in shock, but feel Gerry's presence everywhere. Just wish we could hug him in person. As Amy said, "You can't hug a photograph." During the following week, we were overwhelmed with all the love that came our way: visitors , food, gift baskets, phone calls and so many donations in Grumpy's memory. It's Christmas day, 2007. Carl prepared a delicious pancake breakfast before heading back to Denver this afternoon. Mark made omelets to order, and then brought in a mini-omelet and said, "This is for Grumpy."

Back to Reality

The Rabbi came over this morning to lead us in the prayers that officially end the shiva (mourning) period. He then told us it's time to get on with our lives and commanded me to go shopping. Well, listen, how can I say no to a man of the cloth? So Ronni, Nicole and I went to Sam's Club. Haven't been anywhere in a while, so it was good to get out. Of course, when I told our pharmacist at Sam's about Gerry, she burst into tears and I had to console her. We watched "Dream Girls" today and still enjoy the picture. I spent a good deal of time with phone calls to Social Security, lawyer, insurance companies, etc. Nurse Ratched will get through it, but this kind of paperwork was Gerry's bailiwick, and I have to learn a lot in a very short period of time.

ONE MORE VISIT

Did a few out-of-the-house chores this morning. It's strange, but good, to start going and doing again. Amy wanted to visit Grumpy one time before heading back to Colorado, so Susi, Ronni, Amy, Nicole and yours truly visited our Gerry this afternoon. The Rabbi said it was fine any time after the seven days of mourning. We probably would have done it anyway. Couldn't help but smile at the location of the cemetery. It's in Florida, NY. So Gerry ended up in Florida, albeit not the lala land he loved, but the countryside he loved. And he's just 15 minutes from our house.

A MOVIE!

Today we all went to the movies (my first movie in months!). We saw "Enchanted" and loved every minute of it, especially when the leading lady gets transported to New York City, sees a very little man on the street and says, "Grumpy!" We knew Gerry was with us.

What Now?

Amy and Ryan left today, Ronni left yesterday, and
the house has suddenly become very quiet. My first
reaction was to be devastated and non-accepting.
The thought of never seeing Gerry again was too
hard to handle. After a few months, however, a light
bulb went off in my head. I found a way to deal with
this overwhelming sadness. I just go a day at a time.
I won't see Gerry today. Tomorrow is another day.
Just by taking it a day at a time makes it much more
bearable. And during this process, I can find the joys
in every-day life while remembering the joys of my life
with my Gerry. Received a phone call from someone
from Hospice. I was not interested in group or phone
therapy, and almost hung up, but I decided to be civil
and chat for a few minutes. Rockland County came up
in the conversation, and I mentioned that I graduated
from Spring Valley High School. The Hospice caller
turned out to be somebody I knew 60 years ago. In
fact, I graduated with her sister Judy. The caller was
Elaine Green Allen, and the more we talked, the more
we found common friends and memories. Have been
friends ever since, and we joke about getting together
for lunch...a date that is not a visit to a doctor's office!
I've also joined her weekly card game with the "girls."
We talk, nosh for 4-5 hours and then break for
dinner. I have renamed our group the OCAK
Association, which stands for "Orange County
Alta Kocker" Association.

THE UNVEILING

Since December can be so unpredictable weather-wise, we decided to have the unveiling of Gerry's stone in late August. Traditionally, you leave a little stone on the headstone whenever you visit a grave site. We decided to do something different. Everyone in the family decorated a stone, hand-painting sayings and designs. Rabbi Stemler conducted the service and family and friends all placed their special stones around Grumpy's grave, wishing him a personal farewell. We ordered a double headstone, and Gerry's side had beautiful words etched into it. Since my side was empty, I put a yellow sticky on the blank marble that said,"To Be Announced."

I had one last chance for a song at a Feldman gathering, so I wrote some lyrics (with apologies to Little Mermaid):

We all remember that Gerry Boy...
When he walked in a room, we were filled with joy.
We all remember that Gerry Guy...
Who we miss more and more as days go by.
We miss his warmth, we miss his smile,
We miss his laugh, his wisdom, his style.
And we agree he'll always be part of our world.

It's been more than two years now, and we're all still adjusting. I had my knee replaced... first serious operation without Gerry at my side. But one has to keep going. One has to keep doing. One has to keep busy. Who knows? I may even write a book!

ACKNOWLEDGMENTS

Thanks to brother-in-law Stanley for calling up and saying
"write a book."
To sister-in-law Dolores for writing a 5-star review
via e-mail.
To Susan, Ronni and Amy for their input, their forwards,
encouragement, and their love.
To Mark, Matt and Carl...the world's best sons-in-law.
To Nicole, my graphic arts granddaughter, who designed
this memoir.
To Andrea, for keeping me grounded by calling me
an old poop, and for creating the video promo for the book.
To Eric and Scott for the smiles and the hugs and the caring.
To Ryan for interviewing me as his favorite author in a
school project.
To Joel, Diane and the whole Schatz family for always
being there for me.
To the Feldman gang for the support, visits,
and phone calls.
And thanks to everyone mentioned in this memoir,
and everyone I forgot to mention. You are all so important to
the Audrey and Gerry story, and I love you all.

A very special mention to caringbridge.org. Through
this wonderful website, I was able to keep in touch with
family and friends during a very difficult time.

A portion of the proceeds will be donated to
caringbridge.org, Hospice of Orange and Sullivan
Counties, and to the MHE Coalition.

AUDREY FELDMAN grew up in Spring Valley, NY and attended NYU (attended is another word for did not graduate). She met her one and only Gerry in 1950, they were married in 1951 and produced three beautiful daughters: Susan, Ronni and Amy. She worked as a copywriter and PR director for a wall covering company, and then became art director for a lingerie company that had licenses for the major cartoon characters. During this time she was also a lyricist in Lehman Engel's BMI Workshop, working with composer Don Freeberg. Known for her wicked sense of humor, Audrey's happiest moments are those spent with her family, now consisting of 3 loving daughters, 3 wonderful sons-in-law and 5 incredible grandkids (she also loves adjectives). This book commemorates her life with Gerry, who valiantly fought cancer for eight months - before losing his courageous battle.

GERALD FELDMAN grew up in Brooklyn, NY and went into his family's pajama business. He and Audrey moved many times during their 56-year marriage – from upstate New York to Long Island to Lynchburg, Virginia to Yonkers to Hartsdale to New Jersey and finally, to Delray Beach, Florida. After a collapse of the family business, Gerry became vice president for a major lingerie firm in Manhattan. When the kids were young, he bought a tent, and camping was vacation time for many years. After moving to New Jersey, Captain Gerry traded the tent in for a boat, and many summers were spent cruising on Barnegat Bay (or being towed, if First Mate Audrey read the charts wrong). In 2005, the Feldmans moved to Pine Island, NY, into an apartment in daughter Susan's bi-level home. Gerry loved being with his family, and his family loved being with him until the very last good bye.